Commissioning Editor: Ellen Green
Development Editor: Barbara Simmons
Project Manager: Elouise Ball
Design Direction: Stewart Larking

Complementary Medicine

A Guide for Pharmacists

Denise Rankin-Box
BA (Hons), RGN, Dip TD, CertED, MISMA JP
Company Development Manager, DOT Medical

Editor-in-Chief, *Complementary Therapies in Clinical Practice*
Trustee of British Holistic Medical Association

Elizabeth M Williamson
BSc (Pharm), PhD, MRPharmS, FLS
Professor of Pharmacy and Director of Practice,
University of Reading

Editor-in-Chief, *Phytotherapy Research*
Member of the Herbal Drugs Committees for the British
European Pharmacopoeias

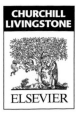

CHURCHILL
LIVINGSTONE

ELSEVIER

Edinburgh   London   New York   Oxford   Philadelphia
St Louis   Sydney   Toronto   2006

CHURCHILL
LIVINGSTONE
ELSEVIER

First published 2006

ISBN 10: 0443 070288
ISBN 13: 9780443 070280

British Library Cataloguing in Publication Data
A catalogue record for this book is available from the British Library

Library of Congress Cataloging in Publication Data
A catalog record for this book is available from the Library of Congress

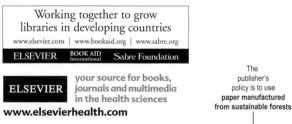

Working together to grow
libraries in developing countries

www.elsevier.com | www.bookaid.org | www.sabre.org

ELSEVIER   BOOK AID International   Sabre Foundation

ELSEVIER   your source for books, journals and multimedia in the health sciences

www.elsevierhealth.com

The publisher's policy is to use paper manufactured from sustainable forests

Printed in China

Contents

Preface and acknowledgements   vii

Why pharmacists need to know about complementary and alternative medicine   ix

1. Complementary therapies, holistic medicine and the placebo effect   1

Complementary therapies encountered by the pharmacist   1
    Table 1.1. Summary of complementary therapies and their uses, for quick reference   3
Holistic medicine – what it means in practice   23
The placebo effect   25

2. Herbal medicine, phytotherapy and nutraceuticals   31

Introduction: systems of herbal medicine   31
Western medical herbalism and rational phytotherapy   40
Nutraceuticals   43
Traditional Chinese Medicine (TCM)   45
    Table 2.1. Treatment of disease in TCM according to the yin and yang nature of the disease and the remedy   51
Ayurveda   52
    Table 2.2. Determining the human constitution according to Tridosha   54
    Table 2.3. Effect of different foods on the Tridosha   56
    Table 2.4. Effect on the Tridosha of some herbs   60
Anthroposophical medicine   62
Comments on traditional herbal medicine systems   64
Choosing a herbal or nutraceutical remedy   65
Regulation of herbal medicines in the UK   66

Table 2.5. Therapeutic indications treated by herbal medicines and supplements   70
Table 2.6. Common nutritional and herbal supplements: a summary of their uses, doses and interactions with prescription and OTC medicines   74

3. Homeopathy and aromatherapy   123

Introduction   123
Homeopathy   127
Aromatherapy   160
   Table 3.1. Some popular homeopathic remedies suitable for pharmacist recommendation or patient self-selection: symptom picture and indications   140
   Table 3.2. Common complaints and homeopathic remedies to choose from   149
   Table 3.3. Homeopathy: external applications   159
   Table 3.4. Pharmacological activities of selected essential oils   161
   Table 3.5. Aromatherapy: Therapeutic indications for popular oils   173

4. Physical therapies   175

Introduction   175
Acupuncture and acupressure   178
Chiropractic   185
Massage   189
Naturopathy   196
Osteopathy   200
Reflexology   205
Shiatsu   211
   Table 4.1. Example of factors contributing to shiatsu diagnosis   214

5. Emotional and psychological therapies   217

Introduction   217
Bach Flower Remedies   219
   Table 5.1. Bach's classification of emotional states and appropriate remedies   220

Table 5.2. Specific flower remedy and indicated
  emotional state   221
Healing   224
Hypnotherapy   230
Music therapy   236

Appendices   241

1. Website information   241
2. Glossary   249
3. Qualification abbreviations   259
4. Normal blood values   267

Index   269

Preface and acknowledgements

This is the first time that we have embarked upon a book together. The whole process has been very enjoyable even though we had to weave our way through respective work and family commitments as well as Liz taking up a new position as Chair of Pharmacy and Director of Practice at the University of Reading.

Many thanks indeed to Elsevier and in particular to Ellen Green, who initiated this venture, and Barbara Simmons, who has remained an enthusiastic and supportive editorial advisor throughout this project.

Our thanks also to our families, Ian, Carla and Felicity, and Paul, Catriona and Olivia, for their patience.

We hope this book will be well used and become an invaluable tool for pharmacists wishing to know more about complementary and alternative medicine.

DRB   2006
EMW

Why pharmacists need to know about complementary and alternative medicine

WHAT IS COMPLEMENTARY AND ALTERNATIVE MEDICINE (CAM) AND WHAT IS THE EXTENT OF ITS USE?

A working definition of *complementary medicine* is 'diagnosis, treatment and/or prevention, which complements mainstream medicine by contributing to a common whole, by satisfying a demand not met by orthodoxy or by diversifying the conceptual framework of medicine' (Ernst 2004). *Alternative medicine* is an older term used to contrast this approach with conventional medicine, and as it is difficult to distinguish the two meaningfully, it is usual to put them together as complementary and alternative medicine or CAM. This term will be used in this book for convenience.

CAM is no longer the province of people with alternative lifestyles or unusual religions; it is commonly used by the general population, including many doctors, pharmacists and nurses. In fact, in 2000–2001, about 20% of the general population used some form of CAM, and this is increasing. As Ernst (2004) points out, this figure only applies to the *general* population, not the *patient* population, in whom he estimates the use can rise to close to 100%. This figure also applies to pharmacists: in a survey of 420 pharmacists at an international conference, 84% reported having tried some form of CAM themselves (Koh et al 2003). So pharmacists are not, as often thought, antagonistic towards CAM; they take it themselves, recommend it and, of course, sell it (there is also the small matter of the high profit margin on supplements).

The term CAM also includes traditional medicine systems such as Traditional Chinese Medicine (TCM) and Ayurveda, which are routinely used by some ethnic populations who do not consider them to be 'alternative' at all. Outside these ethnic groups, such therapies are considered to be CAM and the fact that they are seen as exotic can increase their popularity. However, any remedy given, whether herbal, mineral or animal, is a drug with the same potential as any other. It can have a therapeutic effect, produce an adverse reaction, and interact with conventional treatment. This is where the pharmacist comes into the equation, as outlined below, and why relevant information is needed to protect the patient.

WHY PHARMACISTS NEED TO KNOW ABOUT CAM: HOW TO USE THIS BOOK

The love affair between the public and CAM shows no signs of abating and there is a huge variety of CAM therapies available, ranging from the plausible and evidence based to the downright implausible and even fraudulent. Unfortunately, there is also a corresponding lack of expertise amongst pharmacists, as with the medical and nursing professions, due mainly to inadequacies in their education and training, which makes many feel uncomfortable when dealing with CAM. The purpose of this book is therefore to act as a source of information and a reference for the busy pharmacist at work, when confronted by a query regarding CAM which demands an immediate (or fairly quick, at least!) answer. It aims to answer these sorts of questions relating to the patient:

- What is the therapy about?
- Will it work for me?
- Is it suitable and safe for me?
- Where can I get more information?

It aims to give a concise outline of each therapy commonly encountered in Western community or hospital pharmacy, but one which is sufficiently detailed to enable pharmacists to exercise their professional judgement as to the suitability of a particular treatment for an individual patient. It does not aim to give an in-depth analysis of the philosophy behind the therapy or a moralistic view as to whether pharmacists should recommend it (this depends on the patient and the circumstances) or dictate a course of action for pharmacists.

The pharmacist may encounter queries about CAM in several ways:

- A regular patient, already on conventional treatment, asks for advice about *adding* a CAM to their existing regime.
- The patient wants to take a CAM *instead* of prescription medicine.
- The prescriber is not happy about a patient self-medicating with CAM, but can accept the idea *if* he or she knows it is unlikely to cause problems.
- The prescriber finds a CAM is actually helping a patient and wants to know how and why, and if it is safe to continue.
- A patient wants to take a supplement perceived to be harmless, in order to maintain health.

All of these are encountered regularly in the pharmacy.

Pharmacists are the nation's 'guardians' of medicines. They generally know more about the action and safety of drugs than any other healthcare professional (HCP), they are easily accessible on the high street for advice without an appointment (or a fee) and they are the only HCPs who encounter patients purchasing CAM products whilst picking up their conventional medicines. They may be approached by patients who are reluctant to consult their GP for fear of disapproval or they may need to intervene when a customer tries to purchase a remedy which is unsuitable for him or her, a situation obvious to the pharmacist because of prior knowledge of the patient's condition and existing treatment regime.

However, there is sometimes a perception that pharmacists do not know much about CAM, and the ubiquity of health food shops, with their plethora of exciting products promising anything and everything, can easily tempt the patient away from the 'scientist in the high street' to the untrained sales assistant down the road. Recent scare stories in the media about the dangers of some CAM therapies, and increased education for HCPs, have helped to encourage patients back to the pharmacy for advice on such therapies, but there is still a long way to go. If strategies using the expertise of pharmacists are to succeed, then the pharmacist needs to have the necessary skills and information. It is illogical for pharmacists only to be educated in the use of a limited range of drugs, which are perceived by the medical establishment to be 'acceptable', but not have anything to do with those the public actually wants to take and is already taking in vast amounts.

On encountering a query, the pharmacist can turn to the appropriate section of this book for a quick summary of the advantages and disadvantages of a specific CAM; find the indication if so required; check the potential for interaction with conventional drugs, especially with regard to herbal and nutritional supplements; and then, if appropriate, recommend a treatment or direct the patient to a CAM practitioner – or back to their GP in some cases.

CHOOSING A THERAPY: WHICH CAM THERAPIES ARE APPROPRIATE FOR PHARMACISTS TO RECOMMEND?

Guidelines from the World Health Organization (WHO) acknowledge pharmacists as one of the key information providers for alternative medicines, and a good overview of the issues is available on: www.who.int/medicines/library/trm/Consumer.pdf.

A pharmacist can recommend any CAM therapy if he or she feels professionally competent to do so. This does not mean that the pharmacist must necessarily be a qualified CAM practitioner to recommend a certain type of therapy, or that they must even believe in it personally, but that they should be able to match the needs of a patient with aspects of a particular CAM which may suit them. The primary objective, as with all medicine, is to do no harm and hopefully provide some benefit. The pharmacist should also not insult patients' beliefs and traditions by openly decrying them, although this does not mean that the pharmacist should condone the use of obviously dangerous remedies. For example, the Chinese herb *Aristolochia* is a proven toxin and carcinogen and is well documented as being responsible for many deaths: a belief in TCM does not make it any less so but correspondingly, this fact does not mean that *all* TCM is harmful. This kind of sloppy thinking is exactly the same as the patient who embraces an alternative lifestyle which considers all synthetic drugs to be harmful.

Additionally, all CAM is not the same. Many complementary therapies represent systems of medicine, for example acupuncture, homeopathy or herbalism, whereas others may be primarily diagnostic or therapeutic tools such as iridology, biofeedback or massage. These will be dealt with in two sections: the first involves remedies which are ingested or applied (i.e. any herb, nutritional supplement, essential oil, homeopathic medicine, etc.). These are probably the most important for the pharmacist, as an expert on drugs, as they may have the potential to interact with conventional medication. The second section involves non-drug therapies, which may also be of interest to the patient, and from a pharmaceutical viewpoint may be more suitable for someone already on a complicated medication regime.

LEGAL STATUS OF CAM AND PRACTITIONERS: THE VIEW OF THE ROYAL PHARMACEUTICAL SOCIETY OF GREAT BRITAIN (RPSGB)

In the United Kingdom, under common law enshrined in a Royal charter signed by Henry VIII, it is legal for anyone to practise complementary therapies without training, with the exception of osteopathy and chiropractic which are protected by statute. Therapists may not, however, claim to be statutorily registered in professions such as medicine, nursing, pharmacy or dentistry if they are not.

However, with the growth of national bodies seeking to standardize specific therapeutic practice, it is expected that increasing numbers of therapies will seek statutory regulation in the foreseeable future. Against this background, the selection of a therapy for personal or client use can be difficult, as clients need to identify competent practitioners and pharmacists wish to proffer specific advice on CAM. In response to the House of Lords science and technology (subcommittee 111) report, the RPSGB made a number of recommendations including:

- patients should have ready access to professional help in case they require conventional medical management

- the public should be protected from all forms of inappropriate claims and therapies
- there is a need for impartial and objective advice to be made available to the public and to health professionals
- high-quality clinical trials should be conducted into therapies
- each therapy should be the responsibility of a professional body and all practitioners should be registered with the appropriate body
- greater funding should be made available to assess safety and efficacy of therapies
- NHS research should be conducted into patient satisfaction and therapy efficacy
- there should be a registration system for suppliers of Chinese medicines
- there should be licensing of herbal medicines and good manufacturing procedures
- CAM availability in the NHS should be limited to therapies subject to formal approval (adapted from Kayne 2002).

(Also visit the RPSGB website: www.rpsgb.org.uk.)

CONSUMER GUIDANCE WHEN CONSIDERING CAM TREATMENT

As early as 1993, the Royal College of Nursing issued a consumer checklist (developed by the Complementary Therapies in Nursing Special Interest Group – CTINSIG) to assist patients or clients to feel more confident about choosing a therapy and evaluating the competency of a therapist. This is partially reproduced below.

- What are the therapist's qualifications and how long was the training?
- Is the therapist a member of a recognized, registered body with codes of practice?

- Can the therapist provide the address and telephone number of this organization to check?
- Is the therapy available on the NHS?
- Is there written information about a therapy?
- What to expect during a treatment
- What to expect following treatment
- Indications for and contraindications against treatment
- Professional referral to another therapist/therapy more suited to treating a specific problem
- On-call facility for patient concerns
- Can a GP delegate care to the therapist?
- Is this the most appropriate complementary therapy for the particular problem?
- Does the therapist send a letter to the GP advising of any treatment received?
- Can the patient/client claim for the therapy through a private health insurance scheme?
- Are the patient records confidential?
- What is the cost of the treatment?
- How many treatments will be needed (and therefore what is the total cost)?
- What insurance cover does the therapist have?
- Is there knowledge of underlying pathology?
- Does the therapist communicate issues to the patient's general practitioner?

PROFESSIONAL REGISTERING BODIES

The professional organizations for different therapies continue to evolve. Current lists can be most effectively obtained through the Internet and key websites are offered in this book. However, the list is not exhaustive and in addition it may be helpful to log onto the British Holistic Medical Association (BHMA) and the Prince of Wales Foundation for Integrated Health (POWFIH; see Appendix 1). Some of the abbreviations used by practitioners and registering bodies are given in Appendix 3.

EVIDENCE – OR LACK OF IT – FOR EFFICACY OF COMPLEMENTARY MEDICINE

It is inescapable that there is a lack of research into CAM, a situation accepted by the RPSGB (see guidelines above). This does not deter sections of the public and some may actually consider this as a positive factor, being motivated by antipathy to the medical establishment. The fact remains that many ordinary consumers and patients are registering their opinions and needs with their purchasing power; it is arrogant to dismiss them all as idiots. As shown previously, the HCP with the greatest knowledge of drugs – the pharmacist – often takes CAM in his or her stride and consumes its products! (Koh et al 2003)

Like guns and knives, drugs are powerful tools but they are inanimate objects and require human authority and judgement for proper usage. The lack of research in CAM not only provides a rationale for *not* using these medicines more widely, but the small amount of research that does exist also uncovers a worrying situation in which undeserved criticism (which would never be accepted in conventional medicine) is accepted in CAM. Another frequent complaint about research in CAM is that it is less rigorous than that of conventional medicine; this is undoubtedly true but the evidence shows that the opposite may equally apply. As an example, a recent study showed that different standards were applied to the evaluation of St John's wort as an antidepressant (Kirsch 2003). In general, the efficacy of antidepressant medication is thought to be well established, whereas that of *Hypericum* (St John's wort) is considered doubtful. However, the available data showed that St John's wort and conventional antidepressants are *equally effective* (or ineffective) and that different standards are being applied to evaluate the two types of treatment. Many CAM therapists ruefully admit that while anecdotal evidence is definitely unacceptable in proving efficacy, it appears to be very acceptable for demonstrating toxicity!

Pharmacists are being asked, and are expected to know how, to counsel the patient in these matters. There is no solution except for as much evidence as possible to be put in the public domain, and for practitioners to exercise their professional judgement when it comes to advising the patient of their options and warning them of any possible problems.

SUMMARY

Choosing a complementary therapy entails a thorough investigation of potential benefits as well as contraindications of treatment and the potential for CAM treatment–drug interactions. The pharmacist is ideally placed to fulfil this function once equipped with the relevant information and authority. In the area of consumer guidance, consideration of how to evaluate the effectiveness of the complementary intervention must be taken into account. Those who have used complementary therapies for themselves and for their client group usually recommend proceeding with caution. The pharmacist should consider why and whether a therapy is needed, critically evaluate the potential benefits or contraindications regarding the use of a therapy, and then he or she can objectively appraise the evidence underpinning a therapy.

References and Further Reading

Ernst E 2004 Complementary medicine pharmacist? Pharmaceutical Journal 273:197–198.

Kayne SB 2002 Complementary therapies for pharmacists. Pharmaceutical Press, London.

Kirsch I 2003 St John's wort, conventional medicine and placebo: an egregious double standard. Complementary Therapies in Medicine 11(3):193–195.

Koh H-L, Teo H, Ng H-L 2003 Pharmacists' patterns of use, knowledge, and attitudes to complementary and alternative medicine. Journal of Alternative and Complementary Medicine 9:51–63.

CHAPTER 1

Complementary therapies, holistic medicine and the placebo effect

COMPLEMENTARY THERAPIES ENCOUNTERED BY THE PHARMACIST

Pharmacists are encountering complementary therapies with increasing frequency these days, especially those that could loosely be considered as 'pharmacological therapies'. Many people also tend to assume that a substance that is ingested may interact with their prescription medication and this is probably the single most important reason why pharmacists need to know about CAM.

The pharmacist has to be aware of the potential of substances to interact with prescription medicines despite the lack of published information, a problem we have tried to address in the section on herbal medicines and nutritional supplements. Pharmacists are also in an ideal position to advise the general public about a wide range of preparations. Today, however, they may also be asked about non-pharmacological therapies, such as hypnotherapy, massage, osteopathy or chiropractic, and the extent to which these therapies may augment conventional treatment or provide a *competent* alternative therapeutic approach. An erroneous but popular assumption is that 'natural' therapies are harmless and this has been a powerful marketing tool. Many complementary and alternative medicine (CAM) therapies have a limited research basis and many are still unregulated. In addition, limited funding to assess therapeutic efficacy and safety continues to affect both claims and advice given to the public.

2

It is apparent that little evidence exists concerning the safety or harm associated with particular therapies, either alone or when combined with pharmaceutical preparations. (It is also necessary to note that allopathic medicine does not present a unified body of competent research either and there are still many aspects of clinical practice sadly lacking in competent research studies.) It is therefore a question of balance and of objectively reviewing the research and literature to date in order to offer best advice to the public. It is hoped that this book goes some way to bridging the interface between pharmacists and the general public in the field of CAM.

Classification of CAM can be difficult. Many 'pharmacological therapies' usually involve the administration of a herbal or nutritional product (i.e. a herbal medicine or nutraceutical supplement). These may include Traditional Chinese Medicine (TCM), Ayurveda, application of essential oils (aromatherapy), preparations used in homoeopathy (even though the concentration of drug is below the therapeutic – or even measurable – threshold) or Bach Flower Remedies.

This book aims to inform the pharmacist of common ailments where CAM has been shown to be effective and offers 'at-a-glance' tables to use when responding to queries from the general public. We have also designed a quick reference to the various common types of CAM, with a brief summary of their indications and contraindications, presented in Table 1.1. Some of the therapies included in the table are not dealt with in detail in the text, either because they are a subsidiary part of another therapy (as with reiki, which can be considered a form of 'healing', q.v.), they are therapies rarely encountered by pharmacists (e.g. art therapy or humour and laughter therapy – except involuntarily sometimes!) or because they are too belief based (as opposed to evidence based) for even the most open-minded or 'alternative' pharmacist to subscribe to at present (e.g. crystal therapy, geopathic stress).

Table 1.1 Summary of complementary therapies and their uses, for quick reference (*therapies dealt with in detail)

Therapy	Description	Suggested indications	Contraindications
Acupuncture*	Latin *acus* (needle) and *punctura* (puncture). An ancient form of healthcare practice and medicine which aims to treat illness and maintain health through stimulation of the body's self-healing powers. May involve use of fine needles to stimulate or unblock energy (Qi) flow around the body, herbs, moxibustion, diet and exercise in order to restore harmony, energy balance and maintain health in the body	Back pain Drug dependency Osteoarthritis Insomnia Nausea and vomiting Migraine and headache Weight loss Stroke GI disorders Nausea and vomiting in pregnancy Pregnancy and cervical ripening ENT conditions Cerebral activation Correction of breech presentation Activation of neutrophils	Untrained use of needles, leading to bleeding and pneumothorax (Ernst 2001, Rampes & James 1995) Electrical stimulation of needles may be contraindicated in those with, for example, implantable gastric stimulation (obesity treatment) or heart pacemakers Caution in pregnancy. No absolute contraindications for pregnancy but moxibustion is not recommended and avoidance of specific points during first and second trimesters. Some data to suggest acupuncture by qualified practitioner to treat nausea and vomiting in pregnancy is safe Resterilized needles – potential infection

3

Therapy	Description	Suggested indications	Contraindications
Alexander Technique (AT)	The use of conscious posture and breathing pattern modification to enhance health and well-being. AT is based upon the premise that poor body posture can contribute towards ill health and chronic pain	Improvement of posture Breathing Temporomandibular joint (TMJ) problems Voice projection Some forms of back pain Flexibility Depression Learning difficulties	None known
Anthroposophical Medicine*	Perception of health and disease wherein the soul and spirit are said to affect health. It is believed that there are four manifestations of the body and three systems by which they can function. Approach developed by Rudolf Steiner who claimed health is maintained when the three systems are in harmony	Philosophical and lifestyle approach	None Known

5

Aromatherapy*	Therapeutic use of essential oils derived from plants and flowers. These may be inhaled, ingested (rarely) or combined with carrier oil for application through skin massage	See section on aromatherapy in Chapter 3 Relief of anxiety Insomnia Hypertension Bronchitis Alopecia areata Some skin infections Pain management IBS	See section on aromatherapy in Chapter 3 Drug interactions with certain oils or concentrations
Art Therapy	The therapeutic use of art, drawing, painting or sculpting to facilitate emotional expression and mood enhancement. Sculpture and modelling may be used in certain psychiatric settings as a form of expressionism or, for example, to develop concentration	Anxiety Displacement therapy Associative psychological problems Communication Autism Stress management Relaxation	In psychotherapy – monitoring of therapy

6

Therapy	Description	Suggested indications	Contraindications
Autogenic Training	A psycho-physiological therapy combining relaxation and self-hypnosis in order to train an individual to enter a relaxed receptive state, through which to facilitate mental and physical homeostasis (rebalancing)	Deep relaxation Stress reduction Pain management Phobia Chronic pain Anxiety Bowel disorders IBS Hypertension	Severe mental or personality disorders
Ayurveda*	An indigenous form of Indian medicine based on an ancient system of balance and harmony epitomized by the *Tridosha*; uses traditional formulae and mixtures of herbs and minerals, with a great emphasis on cleansing the system. *Ayur* means life or longevity and *veda* means knowledge. Disease is considered to be an imbalance and treatment aims to restore equilibrium. Ayurvedic medicine can involve a range of procedures including nutrition, exercise, yoga and herbal medicines. In Pakistan it is referred to as unani-tibb or unani. *Related techniques:* herbalism, unani-tibb	System of healthcare/lifestyle	May vary depending upon combination adopted; see section on Ayurveda in Chapter 2

Bach Flower Remedies*	The use of distilled essences of wild flowers taken diluted in water or spirit or as a lotion. Based on the premise that disease is directly related to temperament; thus remedies treat anxiety, insomnia or disharmony. Examples include Olive to promote renewal and regeneration, Agrimony to encourage self-acceptance and joy	Mild emotional and psychological disturbances	None reported. No research evidence of efficacy
Biofeedback	A method of operant conditioning whereby an individual learns to control otherwise involuntary body functions such as heart rate, blood pressure, headaches, insomnia	Asthma Hypertension Headache Pain management Neuromuscular problems (e.g. after stroke) Multiple sclerosis Peripheral vascular disorders Relaxation Migraine Migraine in children Phobia	Certain psychiatric disorders Dementia Alzheimer's Hypotension Seizure disorders

Therapy	Description	Suggested indications	Contraindications
Bowen Technique	Gentle soft tissue manipulation. May be used for stress relief, anxiety. *Related techniques:* massage, shiatsu	See related techniques	See related techniques
Chiropractic	Specializes in the diagnosis and treatment of mechanical disorders of joints and their effects on the nervous system. Chiropractic employs a technique of spinal manipulation based upon the theory that problems associated with vertebral alignment may result in neural, muscular or sensory disorders. Realignment of the spine aims to restore normal movement through manipulation	Relief of low back pain Some back and neck pain Migraine Neck dysfunction Cervical manipulation often safer than side effects of NSAIDs	Unskilled manipulation Low risk of adverse reactions with trained personnel Advanced osteoporosis Malignant spinal disease Patients on anticoagulants (greater risk of cerebrovascular accidents) Mild initial discomfort Arteriosclerosis Traumatic injuries
Colour Therapy	The use of colour in lighting, paints or materials to help ameliorate physical and psychological problems. Said to relate to the 7 main energy centres (chakras) of the body	Colour has an effect upon perception and psychological mood	Strobe lights may induce seizures Bright lights may affect eyesight

Counselling	A repertoire of verbal and non-verbal communication skills employed to promote psychological well-being in order to help clients to identify and clarify life experiences or problems and to support them	Communication Problem identification	In healthcare, formal counselling should only be undertaken by trained counsellors Requirement to define therapeutic boundaries and for effective management of issues to be raised
Crystal Therapy	The belief that minerals and rocks possess therapeutic forms of energy that can be harnessed to promote well-being. For example, crystal promotes harmony; malachite reduces inflammation; amber lifts burdens; coral protects one's emotional foundation. *Related techniques: stone therapy, colour therapy*	Similar to colour therapy Relaxation Colours linked to chakras	None known No research evidence of efficacy

Therapy	Description	Suggested indications	Contraindications
Healing*	Therapeutic form of energy exchange based upon a cause-and-effect relationship between a healer's conscious intention to heal and subsequent improvement in client symptoms and physical and psychological well-being. Term may also be used generically to describe specific 'healing' practices. *Related techniques: therapeutic touch, non-contact touch, spiritual healing, laying on of hands, meditation, reiki*	Health and well-being Some wound healing Anxiety Insomnia Some forms of pain See section on healing in Chapter 5	None known Little research evidence of efficacy
Herbal Medicine*	The use of decoctions of herb and plant material by trained practitioners to facilitate healing and health. Subcategories include botanical medicine, Chinese herbalism, Ayurveda, kampo, phytotherapy, rational phytotherapy	System of medicine See Chapter 2	Inappropriate herbal prescriptions Drug/herb interaction Inappropriate dosage Side effects of medication See Chapter 2

Homeopathy	A very popular system of medicine based upon the Law of Similars (let like be treated with like). Affectivity is obtained through a process of dilution during which extracts from natural sources such as plants and minerals are diluted many times. At each dilution the mixture is sucussed (vigorously shaken). Homeopaths believe succussion enhances the potency of dilution. Homeopathic products include liquid, pill and tablet forms. *Related techniques: bioemic medicine, isopathy, tautopathy*	See section on homeopathy in Chapter 3	Few known; some anecdotal reports of abreaction. Evidence of efficacy sparse and conflicting
Geopathic Stress	Based on a theory that energies emanate from the earth, manifesting through stress or ley ines, which may affect general health and well-being	Diagnostic tool	No conclusive evidence to support diagnostic properties
Hara Diagnosis	A form of diagnosis used in shiatsu and a number of Eastern cultures, involving gentle palpation of the abdominal region. In shiatsu the hara is referred to as the *tandien*, the centre of balance and gravity	Diagnostic tool	Untrained abdominal palpation. No conclusive evidence to support diagnostic properties

Therapy	Description	Suggested indications	Contraindications
Humour and Laughter Therapy	A psychological intervention based upon humour or an amusing intervention designed to be of benefit to the patient. Can be effective in increasing cortisol levels and pain reduction. *Related techniques: displacement therapy, visualization, hypnosis*	Stimulation of immune system Eosinophil enhancement Relaxation Health and well-being	None known
Hypnotherapy*	The deliberate use of the trance state to effect change in the conscious (e.g. breathing) and/or autonomic nervous system (gut peristalsis, blood pressure). A principle of hypnosis is that the individual is in control of their trance state and not the hypnotist. Thus hypnosis is fundamentally self-hypnosis with the therapist acting as a facilitator. *Related techniques: visualization, biofeedback, meditation*	Anxiety Stress management Pain relief Trauma Phobia Hypotension IBS Nausea Emesis in chemotherapy Paediatric pain management Weight loss (obesity)	Psychosis Some personality disorders

| Iridology | A diagnostic tool based on the assumption that examination of the iris can indicate the general status of internal organs | Diagnostic tool | No conclusive research evidence to support iridology as a diagnostic tool |
| Kinesiology | A therapy based on traditional acupuncture theory to determine structural or chemical dysfunction. It is believed that such dysfunction is associated with secondary muscle imbalance. Treatment occurs through manipulation of the cranium and body joints. May also include aspects of other therapies | Diagnostic tool | No conclusive research evidence to support kinesiology as a diagnostic tool |

Therapy	Description	Suggested indications	Contraindications
Massage*	The conscious, deliberate and often formalized use of soft tissue manipulation using pressure, light kneading or traction to promote relaxation and well-being. *Related techniques: Swedish massage, biomassage, shiatsu, aromatherapy, reflexology, Indian head massage, reiki*	Chronic constipation Back massage – elderly institutionalized patients Insomnia Fibromyalgia Low back pain Pain Anxiety Muscular tension and fatigue Improved local and distant lymphatic circulation Enhanced blood circulation Cancer patients (metastases not caused or spread by gentle surface massage, McNamara 1993) HIV/AIDS – loss of weight and/or Kaposi's sarcoma may make massage uncomfortable unless gentle touch and extra lubricant are used	Deep vein thrombosis Burns Skin infections, open wounds Advanced osteoporosis Extremes of body temperature Acute, undiagnosed back pain Fractures – direct massage Unexplained lumps and bumps – should be diagnosed before massage Unstable pregnancy –massage should not be given to the abdomen, legs and feet for the first trimester Chronic fatigue syndrome – patients only tolerate short treatments when the syndrome is active Dementia and psychosis

Music Therapy*	The use of music in order to enhance, improve and maintain a therapeutic effect for physical and psychological well-being	Enhanced spatial awareness with certain types of music Anxiety and uncertainty Reduced neonatal hospital stay Alternative channel of communication for, e.g., autistic children, ADHD Enhanced survival – music and social/cultural activities Enhanced recall in patients with dementia Reduction of pain and anxiety in hospital setting	Choice of music critical Music preferences influenced by culture, age, medical condition (e.g. pain relief, relaxation, coordination) Increased memory recall may initiate negative as well as positive memories
Naturopathy*	A multidisciplinary approach to healthcare founded on a belief in the power of the body to heal itself	Wide range of therapeutic approaches Central tenets of diet, nutrition and exercise to promote health synergy See also indications for other therapies	Safety, efficacy, cost-effectiveness of naturopathy not well documented Due to the basic premise underpinning naturopathy, other therapies may be used after careful consideration; thus contraindications of other therapies should be referred to Excessive heating or cooling of the body should be avoided in weak patients, pregnancy, liver or kidney disorders

16

Therapy	Description	Suggested indications	Contraindications
Neurolinguistic Programming	The use of learnt behavioural strategies and changes to thought patterns to assist problem solving. Effective for anxiety, stress and personal development. *Related techniques: hypnosis, meditation, relaxation, imagery*	Anxiety Stress Psychological problems	See also hypnosis Certain psychological problems
Nutraceuticals*	Supplementation of the diet with natural products made from foods, to maintain health, control or prevent symptoms of disease or certain regenerative disorders related to ageing. *Related techniques: diet, naturopathy*	Healthy diet balance and maintenance; see section in Chapter 2	Young children should be referred to doctor Some allergic skin reactions have been reported Should not be used as a substitute for good nutrition and diet
Nutritional Therapy	Based on the assumption that the state of one's health is directly contingent upon what is eaten. Nutritional therapy focuses upon the effects certain foods have on health and illness. *Related techniques: diet, nutraceuticals*	Relationship between diet and health	Monitoring of specific dietary intolerances and allergies

Osteopathy*	A system of manual medicine concerned with mechanical, functional and postural treatment. Osteopathy involves manipulation of joints and spinal vertebrae aimed at resolving mechanical problems of the body. Osteopaths believe that the central role of the physician is to facilitate self-healing	Joint and mobility restrictions Low back pain Mobility problems	Osteoporosis Spinal trauma Open wounds Broken bones Infections See also Chiropractic
Placebo Therapy*	The administration of a placebo (an inert substance or intervention) in order to initiate a physiological or psychological response	See introductory section	Should only be used in certain carefully considered circumstances for ethical reasons
Qi-Gong	A branch of Chinese medicine integrating exercise, self-massage, structured movements and meditation to enhance Qi energy. *Related techniques: Tai Chi, shiatsu, reiki*	General health promotion See also Tai Chi	None clearly identified

Therapy	Description	Suggested indications	Contraindications
Reflexology*	A treatment which applies varying degrees of pressure, commonly to the hands and feet, to promote health and well-being. Based upon the premise that the internal organs of the body are mapped out on the surface of the hands and feet. Treatment of internal organs occurs through gentle pressure to specific areas of the hands or feet; a change can be effected elsewhere in the body through 'reflexes' or 'zones' that run along the body terminating in the hands or feet. *Related techniques: massage, shiatsu, reiki*	Relaxation Insomnia Non-specific low back pain Anxiety	Not recommended during first trimester of pregnancy
Reiki	Japanese healing discipline derived from the Usui natural healing system (also known as Usui shiki ryoko) involving the laying on of hands. *Rei* means 'universal', *'ki'* means 'life force energy'	Relaxation Calm	None known

| Relaxation* | A state of altered consciousness characterized by the release of muscular tension, anxiety and stress. Can also elicit a relaxation response of the autonomic nervous system. Process involves progressive muscular relaxation. Relaxation exercises are frequently incorporated into healthcare practice and antenatal care. *Related techniques: visual guided imagery, autogenic therapy, hypnosis, biofeedback, yoga, meditation* | Hypertension
Insomnia
Arthritis
Pain management
Stress management
Relief of menopausal symptoms
Oncology
Depression
Strengthen immune system
Pain management – increased efficiency when used with visualization
Reduction in side effects of nausea and vomiting caused by radiotherapy or chemotherapy
Decreased postoperative
Development of analgesia
Positive attitude
Panic attacks | Difficulty acquiring skill
Sustaining concentration required to elicit relaxation response
Dyspnoea
Psychosis
Allergic or other adverse reactions may result if certain visualization triggers are activated, e.g. picturing a corn field for a patient with hay fever
Rarely, may exacerbate depressive state |

Therapy	Description	Suggested indications	Contraindications
Shiatsu*	Literally means 'finger pressure'. A physical therapy grounded in Japanese culture based upon the same premise as acupuncture. Rather than using fine needles to stimulate and harmonize Qi energy flow around the body, Shiatsu practitioners direct pressure to key points (*tsubos*) to promote health and well-being. *Related techniques: acupuncture, moxibustion, reiki, massage*	Relaxation Tired eyes, sinus congestion Constipation Menstrual cramps Motion sickness Nausea Some digestive disorders Tension headaches Postmyocardial infarction nausea and vomiting (PMINV) Pregnancy and childbirth (see also acupuncture) Pain and nausea relief in palliative care	Osteoporosis Burns Broken skin Bruises Direct pressure over varicose veins Low platelet count Fevers Inflammation Swelling Skin infections
Tai Chi	A process of systematic slow martial art movements and physical postures to promote flexibility, focus and harmony	Suppleness Relaxation Breathing	None known

Therapeutic touch (TT)	Described as an energy field interaction between two or more people with the intention to rebalance or repattern the energy field in order to facilitate relaxation and self-healing. See also healing. *Related techniques: healing, spiritual healing, non-touch healing, visualization*	Relaxation Wound healing Anxiety Stimulation of immune system	None known specifically
Traditional Chinese Medicine* (TCM)	Based upon a sophisticated and ancient system of balance and harmony epitomized by yin and yang; uses traditional formulae and mixtures of herbs, plus other non-drug treatment such as acupuncture	Range of approaches within TCM. See also herbal mecicine, massage, acupuncture	See also massage, acupuncture, homeopathy, herbal remedies
Visualization*	Use of imagination and psychological imagery to positively influence health. For example, anxiety reduction, insomnia, panic attacks, management of pain	See relaxation	See relaxation

Therapy	Description	Suggested indications	Contraindications
Yoga	The practice of gentle structured breathing, meditation and stretching exercises to promote flexibility and relaxation. Yoga is derived from the Sanskrit word *yuj* meaning 'to yoke'. The purpose is to join the mind to the body through harmonious breathing, meditation and physical exercise. The main yoga practices used in the West are breath control (*pranayama*), meditation and poses (*asanas*). *Related techniques: Tai Chi, meditation*	Relaxation Maintenance of flexibility and suppleness Beneficial for all ages See also meditation	Osteoporosis During limb muscle injury Known back/vertebral problems

Those therapies in the table which are dealt with in more detail are marked with an asterisk*.

HOLISTIC MEDICINE – WHAT IT MEANS IN PRACTICE

Holism means viewing the patient as a whole person and not just a collection of symptoms, in that all facets of an individual's make-up are afforded consideration when arriving at a diagnosis or treatment regime. Although this is becoming more widely recognized as an essential part of all types of therapy, emphasis upon symptom assessment and management is still the fulcrum of Western medicine. It is only very recently that some basic holistic factors contributing to health (diet, emotional support and the importance of palliative care, for example) have been given greater priority in UK hospitals. Many healthcare professionals (not to mention patients) still perceive a void in healthcare, which has led to many being dissatisfied with conventional medical practice. In fact, one of the reasons why CAM is popular is because of a perceived lack of humanity in the conventional healthcare field.

The 'clinical gaze'

Cognitive and emotional distancing of practitioner from client, common in allopathic medicine, was referred to as 'the clinical gaze'. Health workers were encouraged to leave personal life and emotional responses to clinical encounters at the door of the surgery or hospital. This affected the process of healthcare in a number of ways. The emphasis upon objective treatment made no allowance for therapeutic and empathic care which are particularly human traits and ones that are now recognized as crucial to the healing process. Patients frequently felt unable to express their anxieties or emotional responses to their own or a loved one's clinical condition and felt that they must be stoical and not expressive in any way. This resulted in confused healthcare workers, who were ill equipped to manage emotional aspects of patients' illnesses, and their own feelings about their work and for the patients within their care. The very human desire to care for patients was frequently countermanded by an imperative for objectivity.

This attitude is rejected by most CAM practitioners and the growing social trend towards individualized patient care perceived as central to CAM is embodied by the value afforded to the equal interplay between personal, social and spiritual aspects of humanity upon health and well-being.

In an increasingly technological, socially fragmented environment, complementary therapies have been adopted in part because they legitimize individualized care and touch, and a belief that each one of us is unique and requires personalized medicine.

The 'pharmaceutical gaze'

The ability of the pharmacist to see all aspects of medicines, from their physicochemical and pharmacological properties through to clinical evidence, has been described as 'the pharmaceutical gaze' (Barber 2005). This is now considered to be only one part of being a pharmacist, with the ethical and human side becoming of equal importance; a holistic approach is not the exclusive domain of any specific healthcare group.

Pharmacists, especially those engaged in community pharmacy, generally get to know their patients in much the same way as general practitioners do, and sometimes better, because an appointment is not needed to talk to us, we are almost always available and pharmacists are not perceived to be as 'busy' as a GP. Advertising tells the public to 'ask your pharmacist' so we can hardly complain when they do, and this contact with patients can be one of the most rewarding parts of the job. We hear their personal problems, we watch their children grow up and unfortunately our patients will die; in between, they ask for advice on all kinds of health matters – including CAM.

THE PLACEBO EFFECT

Definitions

The placebo effect is a positive therapeutic outcome that can occur after the administration of an inert substance or intervention by initiating a physiological or psychological response (*placebo* is derived from the Latin meaning 'I please'). A self-healing response may be termed a placebo response. Some authors prefer the term 'belief response' to placebo response, since the effect may be due to the patient's belief and not the 'fake' medicine. There are many examples in the literature and the issue, as it applies to pharmacists, has recently been reviewed by Sturgess (2005).

A 'negative placebo' is often termed a *nocebo*. This occurs when the outcome is the opposite of a placebo effect and is an adverse side effect which may occur after the administration of an inert substance (or intervention). The nocebo effect is often prompted by the suggestion that an unwanted effect may occur and is becoming recognized as a possible factor in adverse drug reactions. Indeed, a nocebo may actually be responsible for some adverse reactions which have erroneously been attributed to drug therapy (Ferreres et al 2004).

In a study of over 600 patients in three different centres in Italy, the overall occurrence of the nocebo effect as a factor in adverse reactions in clinical practice was estimated at 27%. Subjective symptoms (itching, malaise, etc.) were measured and the occurrence was found to be significantly higher in women than in men (Liccardi et al 2004).

Ethical considerations

The placebo effect is often stated as the source of clinical efficacy associated with complementary or alternative medicine. To complicate matters, placebos are sometimes used as a therapy in their own right and it is now known that placebo therapy can result in measurable physiological changes, not to mention clinical outcomes. However, there is much dispute as to whether a placebo should be used as a therapy, rather than just acting as a control in a clinical trial. Ernst (2004) describes the dangers of employing a pure placebo treatment as leading 'straight back to the dark ages of medicine' and suggests that adopting it as a complementary medicine would be 'counterproductive'. He also points out that the placebo effect is too unpredictable to be relied upon.

However, before pharmacists dismiss all use of placebos as either unethical or fraudulent, it would be wise to remember how we deal with our own children. How many parents, after a minor accident, apply an unnecessary plaster or bandage and give their children a treat, some 'medicine' or extra affection? If the placebo effect is indeed unethical, logically we should stop these comforting and harmless practices.

This book therefore attempts to make no moral judgements as to whether pharmacists should recommend or even sell alternative medicines for which no evidence is available (and many of which are also implausible), but to present current opinion, popular belief and evidence where it does exist, so the pharmacist can exercise his or her own professional judgement – as with any other pharmaceutical issue.

A paper by Vrovac (2004), entitled 'Placebos and the Helsinki Declaration – what to do', examines the ethical dilemma posed by knowingly administering a placebo. The Helsinki Declaration is the 'gold standard' (and a directive, not a law) covering how to conduct controlled studies in humans in conformity with ethical principles. It demands that 'the best treatment' be used, which could be taken to mean that it excludes the use of placebos in control groups. However, Vrovac concludes that employment of a placebo is justified when its use does not cause irreversible damage or considerable suffering to the 'well-informed patient'.

A medicolegal case report from the US (Rich 2003) described a situation where an adolescent with migraine headache had a placebo (saline injection) substituted for an opioid (morphine). Although the placebo was effective enough in reducing the headache for the patient to be discharged from hospital, when the mother found out, she filed charges of professional misconduct against almost everyone involved, because of the 'deceptive' use of a placebo (as if it is possible to use a placebo any other way). The medical board declined to take action against the physician and although the case involving the nurse did go to court, it was successfully challenged, illustrating that the ethics of placebo use remain a concern and that although the patient may get better, they may still (in the US at least) sue!

Mechanisms by which placebos and nocebos may act

Placebo drug reactions have recently been studied systematically for efficacy and safety in drug data pooled from randomized, placebo-controlled multicentre studies (Weihrauch 2004). The efficacy of the placebo on clinical symptoms varied according to the therapeutic indication, but it had no effect on laboratory values such as blood glucose in diabetics. This suggests that the use of a placebo may be justified in some types of disease where it is known to be helpful, but *not* instead of effective treatments which are already established, for example in metabolic diseases where it is necessary to alter blood physiological parameters such as cholesterol, glucose, thyroid hormones, etc. to maintain health.

An experiment to investigate whether placebo and nocebo responses could be mediated via modulation of stress (measured by analysing blood levels of cortisol and beta-endorphin) showed that although the *perception* of pain was decreased in the placebo group, this did not actually correlate with cortisol and beta-endorphin levels. In the nocebo group, although the expectation of pain led to an increase in cortisol, neither this expectation nor the increased cortisol had any effect on pain (Johansen et al 2003).

Placebo and nocebo responses are believed to be mediated by both cognitive and conditioning mechanisms, but little is known about their role in different circumstances. Experiments designed to elucidate these mechanisms were carried out on experimental ischaemic arm pain in healthy volunteers and motor performance in Parkinsonian patients, using verbally induced expectations of improvement or worsening of symptoms. These opposing verbal suggestions were also able to completely override a preconditioning procedure (Benedetti et al 2003). The authors suggested that placebo responses are mediated by conditioning when unconscious physiological functions (such as hormonal secretion) are involved, whereas they are mediated by expectation when conscious physiological functions (such as pain and motor performance) are concerned, even though a conditioning procedure was used.

Parkinson's disease (PD) is known to have a significant placebo response rate which is related to dopamine release in the striatum. Expectation is also known to be a very important part of the placebo response and in another study of Parkinsonian patients, the placebo effect was found to be related to the expectation of clinical benefit during treatment with deep brain stimulation (DBS). Patients who had previously experienced DBS had a higher response rate to active treatment and the estimated magnitude of the placebo effect in DBS was equivalent to 39% of the magnitude of the effect of active DBS (de la Fuente-Fernandez 2004). The nature of the disease, as well as other factors, is important, with PD, depression and pain having particularly high placebo response rates. Nicotine replacement therapy in smoking cessation also has a demonstrable placebo effect: regardless of actual treatment, smokers who believed they had received nicotine had a significantly better outcome in one study than those who believed they had received placebo (Dar et al 2005).

Conclusion

Placebo and nocebo responses are well-documented effects, although their incidence is disputed (Hrobjartsson & Gotzsche 2004) and the ethics of administering them, even in placebo-controlled clinical trials, is becoming contentious. From the pharmacist's point of view, there may be a dilemma in advising a patient to take something for which no evidence (or even theory) exists. The practical answer is usually to be tactful and perhaps suggest that 'many people find it effective' or that 'it might be worth a try' rather than challenging the beliefs of the patient and denigrating what may be a favoured and effective medicine *for a particular person.*

References

Barber N 2005 The pharmaceutical gaze – the defining feature of pharmacy? Pharmaceutical Journal 275:78.

Benedetti F, Pollo LA, Lopiano L, Lanotte M, Vighetti S, Rainero I 2003 Conscious expectation and unconscious conditioning in analgesic, motor and hormonal placebo/nocebo responses. Journal of Neuroscience 23(10):4315–4323.

Dar R, Stronguin F, Etter JF 2005 Assigned versus perceived placebo effects in nicotine replacement therapy for smoking reduction in Swiss smokers. Journal of Consulting and Clinical Psychology 73(2):350–353.

de la Fuente-Fernandez R 2004 Uncovering the hidden placebo effect in deep-brain stimulation for Parkinson's disease. Parkinsonism and Related Disorders 10(3):125–127.

Ernst E 2001 The desktop guide to complementary and alternative medicine: an evidence based approach. Mosby, Edinburgh.

Ernst E 2004 Medicine man: the placebo effect might make you feel better, but that doesn't mean it will work for everyone. The Guardian 18 May:11.

Ferreres J, Banos JE, Farre M 2004 Nocebo effect: the other side of placebo. Medicina Clinica 122(13):511–516.

Hrobjartsson A, Gotzsche PC 2004 Is the placebo powerless? Update of a systematic review with 52 new randomized trials comparing placebo with no treatment. Journal of Internal Medicine 256(2):91–100.

Johansen O, Brox J, Flaten MA 2003 Placebo and nocebo responses, cortisol and circulating beta-endorphin. Journal of Psychosomatic Medicine 65(5):786–790.

Liccardi G, Senna G, Russo M et al 2004 Evaluation of the nocebo effect during oral challenge in patients with adverse drug reactions. Journal of Investigational Allergology and Clinical Immunology 14(2):104–107.

McNamara P 1993 Massage for people with cancer. Wandsworth Cancer Support Centre, London.

Rampes H, James R 1995 Complications of acupuncture. Acupuncture in Medicine 8:26–33.

Rich BA 2003 A placebo for the pain: a medico-legal case analysis. Pain Medicine 4(4):366–372.

Sturgess R 2005 Belief: an amazing healing device. Pharmaceutical Journal 274:590–592.

Vrovac B 2004 Placebo and the Helsinki Declaration – what to do? Science and Engineering Ethics 10(1):81–93.

Weihrauch TR 2004 Placebo treatment is effective differently in different diseases – but is it also harmless? Science and Engineering Ethics 10(1):151–155.

CHAPTER 2

Herbal medicine, phytotherapy and nutraceuticals

INTRODUCTION: SYSTEMS OF HERBAL MEDICINE

Herbal and nutritional medicine in the West now encompasses many different traditions, from indigenous folklore to imported Asian systems such as Traditional Chinese Medicine (TCM) and Ayurveda.

Although having a historical basis, it is continually evolving and now also extends to include modern dietary considerations. Most practitioners will use an array of herbal and nutritional supplements depending on their own experience and preferences, and the public are made aware of new (and old) products via the Internet and media. There are, of course, as many types of herbal medicine as there are ethnic groups in a society but the most important systems of herbal medicine include the following.

Traditional (Western) medical herbalism

Use of herbal extracts, teas or other preparations, to traditional formulae. They may be designed for self-medication or prescribed for an individual patient by a practitioner, in a holistic manner.

Rational phytotherapy

May be termed 'evidence-based herbal medicine'. Involves the use of herbal extracts which have been investigated either scientifically or clinically and which are usually administered as a single herb product, processed to give a standardized extract. They are treated in a similar way to conventional medicines – which, in essence, they are, the main difference being that they are of natural origin and contain a complex mixture of phytochemicals as is found within the plant. These products are designed for self-medication but are also prescribed by a practitioner.

Nutraceuticals (functional foods)

The use of items usually found in the diet, often in a more concentrated form, administered not only to rectify omissions in the nutritional quality of the diet but to act as medicines and prevent or treat diseases. The aim of preventing degenerative conditions such as cardiovascular disease is a very popular application of nutraceuticals; this is often termed 'chemoprevention'.

Traditional Chinese Medicine (TCM)

The Chinese equivalent of traditional Western herbalism, although the philosophical basis is much more complex, involving the concepts of 'Qi' and the more familiar yin and yang. It uses herbal extracts, teas or other preparations, again to traditional formulae. TCM is used for self-medication but more often prescribed for an individual patient by a highly trained practitioner.

Ayurveda

The most ancient of all systems of herbal medicines, again with a complicated and holistic philosophical basis, involving the concepts of the Tridosha, 'Vata', 'Pitta' and 'Kapha', and using extracts, teas and some other unique preparations, to traditional formulae. They are also designed for self-medication or prescribed for an individual patient by a practitioner, in a holistic manner.

Anthroposophical Medicine

A perception of health and disease based on the work of Rudolf Steiner, who considered that the soul and spirit affect health. Practitioners use a range of treatments, including diet, massage and prescribed movements (known as eurythmy) and also art therapy, in addition to herbs and minerals. The most important application of anthroposophical medicine, and one which a pharmacist may encounter, is probably mistletoe therapy. However, there are many other products available.

PHARMACEUTICAL ASPECTS OF HERBAL MEDICINES

From the point of view of the pharmacist, the principles behind the different types of herbal therapies may be less important than the effects of natural drugs on the body, and how they may interact with prescribed or over-the-counter (OTC) medicines. The crucial aspect is having enough information to advise patients whether herbal or nutritional supplements are likely to help their condition, how (and for how long) they should be taken, including a suitable trial period, and if they can take them concurrently with prescribed medication or not.

Information on products used in all the above varieties of herbal medicine is collated in Table 2.6 (see p.74) and no distinction is made between them here because there is so much overlap. It must be borne in mind that there are large gaps in our knowledge and this table only represents what is known at present from the published literature. The main reason for the dearth of information regarding efficacy and drug interactions is that traditional medicine is just that: traditional. It derives from folk use, is often passed down by word of mouth and in many cases has not been validated clinically or scientifically. It is complicated by the fact that the herbal medicines used by a society vary according to the natural flora of the region, although there are many common herbs used throughout the world, whose use has been spread by the migration of people taking their medicinal plants and knowledge with them. Additionally, related species, containing similar phytochemicals, are used in different regions of the world according to the habitat of the plant. For example, valerian (*Valeriana* spp) has a long history of use as a sedative in Europe, India, China, Mexico, Africa and elsewhere. The species used are distinct and the constituents may vary somewhat but are still related; however, it is not possible to assume therapeutic equivalence between species without extensive testing.

Apart from the geographical variation in medicinal plant use, there is a lack of scientific evidence even for some of the most widely used herbs, due to the fact that it is difficult to patent anything arising from traditional knowledge, so a herbal or pharmaceutical company cannot recoup the financial outlay needed to provide proof of efficacy. The situation that applies to herb–drug interactions not only involves these factors but is complicated by the lack of reports about them, which is being remedied by initiatives designed to improve reporting of such interactions. Unfortunately, in many cases patients do not consider their herbal and nutritional supplements to be 'drugs' and as such do not mention them to their doctor. Herbal and nutritional products are processed in a variety of ways which affect the composition of the final product and this compounds the issue; one type of product based on the same plant may be more or less safe, efficacious and liable to interactions than another.

Despite the limitations of our knowledge of herbal medicines, it is still necessary to exercise judgement and caution when evaluating these products, and to expand our database of proven effects whenever possible. There is little point in trying to discourage patients from self-medicating with natural medicines as it is part of human nature (and mainly laudable) to try and improve health by exercise, nutritional and other lifestyle methods. Herbal medicines are part of this and are constantly promoted in popular newspaper and magazine articles. It is also a political issue: there is a common perception by some sectors of society that large pharmaceutical companies somehow conspire to suppress the use of herbal medicines for their own financial ends – something for which there is no evidence at all.

These different aspects of the use of herbal medicines are important but to the busy pharmacist, the main problem is the patient who enters either their hospital or community pharmacy, who may be taking a herbal remedy or who would like to, and how to advise them. Pharmacists normally err on the side of caution but even this has its disadvantages: if a patient has been happily taking a supplement for many years and believes it is helping them, they are unlikely (and with justification) to believe the pharmacist who tells them – armed with little evidence but motivated by fear of litigation – that it could be dangerous. This book is aimed at that pharmacist and covers the supplements he or she is most likely to encounter.

However, if the case history is complicated, it may be advisable to recommend that the patient consult an alternative practitioner, who will have more specialist knowledge as well as more time to spend on consultation. There is no doubt that individual attention, not only to treating illness but also assessing lifestyle issues, is an integral part of holistic therapies in general, and the CAM practitioner may be better placed than the busy pharmacist to diagnose and prescribe herbal and nutritional medicines and monitor their use. However, many people take a great interest in CAM (estimated as 30–49% in the US and 20% in the UK) and like to use it themselves and for their family on a basis of self-medication, utilizing knowledge acquired from books, magazines, newspapers, television and radio. So although efficacy of some remedies may be unproven, and indeed the placebo effect may be responsible for at least a part of the effects, it is paramount that the pharmacist can advise on suitability in a non-judgemental fashion (this is not to say in a non-critical way) as the views of the patient must always be respected. If the pharmacist cannot or will not help, the patient may turn to non-expert sources of information with unpredictable results. It must also be mentioned that although some professionals do not consider rational phytotherapy (the evidence-based form of herbal medicine) to be part of CAM, this distinction is rarely appreciated by the public.

Some herbal medicines are also nutrients (e.g. garlic, ginger, turmeric, artichoke) and others (e.g. hawthorn, passiflora, elderflower) contain phytochemicals also common in foods, particularly flavonoids, vitamins and minerals, but in a more concentrated form. It is difficult and not always useful to differentiate between herbs and nutritional supplements, and for this reason they will be dealt with together here. Other herbal remedies (e.g. St John's wort, *Ginkgo biloba*, echinacea) are never normally used as foods, but due to licensing constraints may be sold under food legislation rather than the Medicines Act regulations. Further information on the legal situation can be found later in this chapter.

A very brief outline of the philosophies of different systems of herbal medicine will be given, mainly so the pharmacist has a basic practical knowledge and can explain to the patient what to expect, should they wish to consult a practitioner. The methods by which herbs are prepared for administration (e.g. as herbal teas, fluid extracts, tinctures, etc.) are explained in Box 2.1. Mistletoe therapy is probably the only example of anthroposophical medicine encountered by most pharmacists, as some of the preparations are for injection and are therefore classified as prescription-only medicines (POM).

Box 2.1: Forms of herbal preparations

Herbal teas or infusions

As the name suggests, these are aqueous preparations made by pouring boiling water over finely chopped botanical drugs. Commercially prepared tea bags are available for the most popular herbs, e.g. chamomile, peppermint. Patients often make these at home (this should only be done with very safe herbs as the dose will vary). The usual quantities used for infusion are 500 ml (or 1 pint) of water to 30 g (or 1 oz) of drug. The infusion is then allowed to stand for up to 30 minutes with occasional stirring, and the clear liquid then decanted or strained. Being extemporaneous preparations, made without preservatives, infusions should be taken in divided doses throughout the day of preparation. They are used when the drug to be extracted has a light structure, as with leaves.

Decoctions

These are used for harder materials such as roots and barks, and are made in similar strengths to infusions. Cold water is poured onto the powdered botanical drug, the mixture is heated and allowed to simmer. When cool, the decoction is strained and as with infusions, decoctions should be prepared freshly each day.

Liquid extracts

Liquid extracts provide a more permanent and concentrated formulation. They are prepared by percolation or maceration of the crushed or powdered drug, with water or a mixture of water and alcohol, to produce a liquid extract where a unit of volume represents a unit weight of drug. For example, a 1:1 extract means that the medicinal value of 1 g of drug is contained in 1 ml extract.

Solid extracts

These are prepared by evaporating down either the freshly expressed juices of the herb or liquid extracts produced as explained above. The solvent is evaporated off, leaving a residual extract, which can then be made into tablets or other formulations. These extracts represent a much larger quantity of the drug from which they are prepared than do liquid extracts, tinctures or infusions.

Tinctures

These are liquid preparations using differing strengths of alcohol as their solvent, and so are more permanent preparations. They are particularly suitable for extracting drugs containing resinous and volatile principles. Tinctures are usually made in strengths of 1 in 5, where 5 ml tincture represents the medicinal value of 1 g drug, or 1 in 10, where 10 ml represents 1 g.

Tablets and capsules

These are made in the same way as conventional pharmaceuticals, by mixing herbal extracts or powders with suitable excipients to aid binding and dissolution, then either filling capsules or compressing into tablets.

The quality of herbal and nutritional products

One of the main concerns, and criticisms, of herbal medicine and nutritional supplements regards their safety. Several recent cases of toxicity of herbal products have arisen as a result of contamination or misidentification of plant materials, sometimes accidentally, in other instances deliberately. The lack of regulation has exacerbated these problems and given ammunition to those who wish to deny public access to herbal or other CAM products. It is no more reasonable to label CAM as dangerous because of some fraudulent practitioners, manufacturers or importers than it is to label conventional medicine dangerous since similar problems, including counterfeit medicines and iatrogenic disease, exist here too.

The issue for pharmacists is to decide whether a CAM product is of good quality; otherwise any advice about its use and efficacy is meaningless. For some herbal materials and essential oils, the quality is being addressed by the national authorities (British and European Pharmacopoeia committees) but it can be a problem to distinguish poor products from good ones in the absence of any standards and legal regulation. As with most products and services, good quality does not come cheaply. If *Ginkgo biloba* tablets can be bought over the Internet at £5 for 500, when the brand leader costs £10 for 30, questions need to be asked about the source and quality of the former. There is no answer to this except for the pharmacist to exercise common sense and professional judgement, and maybe point out to the patient that as with so much in life, you get what you pay for.

Western Medical Herbalism and Rational Phytotherapy

> **Principles:** holistic; uses whole extracts of herbs and mixtures of herbs, since these are thought to be synergistic. Rational phytotherapy is a more modern, evidence-based variant but medical herbalism has a very long history and is based on traditional use
>
> **Positive aspects:** increasingly substantiated by recent research; widely accepted by patients; most common herbs are fairly safe; more complicated remedies usually prescribed by herbal practitioner
>
> **Negative aspects:** lack of regulation, little evidence for some treatments; may interact with conventional drugs; adverse drug reactions possible

Herbal medicine in general has a historical basis in Galen's model of 'body humours', which lasted until Culpeper's time and beyond. The humours were blood, black bile, yellow bile and phlegm, each possessing a 'temperament' (hot, cold, dry, damp), and illness was the result of an imbalance in these humours. Herbs had similar properties so for example, a 'cooling' herb such as peppermint would be used to treat a 'hot' condition, such as fever. Medical herbalism today still draws on traditional knowledge but may also be supported by modern diagnoses such as hypertension, hypercholesterolaemia and irritable bowel syndrome. Rational phytotherapy uses standardized products with known concentrations of constituents and there is an increasing emphasis on using evidence from recent randomized controlled clinical trials to support the traditional use of herbal medicines.

Some other features of modern-day herbalism include the following.

- Herbalists select herbs on an individual basis for each patient so even patients with the same physical symptoms may receive different combinations of herbs.

- Herbalists attempt to identify an underlying cause for the illness and to treat this as well, rather than just treating symptoms.
- Herbs are used over a period of time in a gentle manner, to stimulate healing capacity, strengthen bodily systems and correct disturbed body functions. Instant cures are not expected or sought.
- Herbal prescriptions are mixtures, often with at least one component added to 'cleanse the system', 'eliminate toxins' (this usually means a laxative!) or 'stimulate' the circulation.

41

A basic tenet of herbalism is that a whole extract of the herb should be used, e.g. a tincture, herbal tea or pill made from the extract, because the different constituents of a herb act together in a synergistic manner, producing an effect greater than the total contribution of each individual constituent, or because the effects of one constituent reduce the likelihood of adverse effects due to another constituent. It is also believed that some combinations of herbs interact in this way and even if not truly synergistic, this multitarget approach can be termed 'polyvalent action'. There is increasing experimental evidence that this may occur but the science of herbal synergism is still in its infancy (Williamson 2001).

A wide range of disorders can be treated with herbal medicines, although there is concern when serious diseases are treated by CAM. Many practitioners work together with the medical profession to give symptomatic relief and adjunctive therapy to improve quality of life, if not actually cure the patient. The following chronic conditions, which may not be completely relieved by conventional medicine, are prevalent in patients who consult herbalists.

- Digestive and bilious disorders and irritable bowel syndrome

- Hormonal problems in women, such as premenstrual syndrome and menopausal symptoms
- Acne, eczema and other chronic skin conditions
- Intractable pain in inflammatory diseases, arthritis and migraine
- Depression and chronic fatigue syndrome
- Chronic infections such as cystitis and bronchitis

Herbalists' prescriptions

Generally, but not always, a combination of several different herbs is used. Herbalists usually prescribe and dispense herbal medicines as tinctures, blended if necessary, although sometimes more concentrated formulations (fluid extracts) are used. Other oral formulations (tablets, capsules) and topical preparations of herbs may also be prescribed. As long as the actual botanical source(s) of the herbal medicine(s) used is known, the safety and interaction profile (if known) can be obtained from Table 2.6, regardless of whether the remedy was prescribed by a CAM practitioner or bought for self-medication.

Self-medication

Patients should be encouraged to purchase good-quality remedies, if possible from the pharmacy from which they get their prescriptions, so accurate advice can be obtained from the pharmacist who has access to their patient medication records (PMRs). Table 2.6 (p.74) can be used to check the suitability of a product for a particular patient and provides a brief profile of the supplement.

Nutraceuticals

> **Principles:** supplementation of the diet with natural products made from foods, to maintain health, control or prevent symptoms of disease and retard certain degenerative disorders related to ageing
>
> **Positive aspects:** most common nutraceuticals are fairly safe; very fashionable and widely accepted by patients because of their natural origin
>
> **Negative aspects:** lack of regulation; poor quality of some products; may be used by some patients instead of a balanced healthy diet; may (like other foods) interact with conventional drugs

What are nutraceuticals? An overview

Nutraceuticals are sometimes known as 'functional foods' but it is useful for our purposes to distinguish between these terms. A functional food may be defined as 'one that has incorporated into it a component to give it a specific medical or health benefit' whereas a nutraceutical is 'a product produced from food, but presented in a form not usually associated with food (e.g. tablets, capsules)'. They are also described as nutritional supplements or 'phytochemicals', a term that demonstrates their similarity to herbal medicines, and in fact the line dividing them is very blurred, partly because some preparations are both, as discussed earlier. The problem is also exacerbated by the legal situation, where herbal medicines without market authorization are sold under food legislation rather than as medicines.

Functional foods, as defined above, include for example 'bio' yogurts and other fermented milk drinks, which may be designated 'probiotics' and are intended to colonize (or re-colonize) the gut with *Lactobacillus acidophilus* as a general health precaution or to rectify the perceived imbalance produced by antibiotic therapy which can lead to infection with Candida. Many other familiar foods are now fortified or reformulated to give a more 'healthy' alternative: for example, margarines made with plant sterols to reduce blood cholesterol levels; bread made with linseed and soya, as a source of phyto-oestrogens to minimize menopausal symptoms; cereals with added vitamins, and so on. These are considered to be outside the scope of this book, although the phytochemicals they contain are often found in herbal medicines and dietary supplements, and are therefore covered in that respect.

Nutraceuticals may be concentrated extracts of foods and this is where the overlap with herbal medicines is even more pronounced, for example the soya isoflavones, lycopene, beta-carotene and octosanol. Some of these are also known to have chemopreventive effects (against cancer mainly) but there is some doubt as to whether taking isolated compounds in the form of a capsule or other preparation confers the same benefits as a varied diet. Extracts of animal origin are also included, such as chitosan, which is obtained from shellfish, and chondroitin, from cartilage; these are unsuitable for vegetarians but supplements such as creatine, carnitine and other dietary amino acids may be obtained from various other (non-animal) sources. The effects, contra-indications and possible drug interactions of nutraceuticals are included in Table 2.6.

Nutrition proper, the correction of poor diet, control of obesity and dietary management of metabolic illnesses such as diabetes and hypertension are mainly the province of the dietitian. Although pharmacists can and do advise on these subjects, this book is concerned with supplementation and not radical lifestyle advice.

Traditional Chinese Medicine (TCM)

Principles: holistic; based on a sophisticated and ancient system of balance and harmony epitomized by the principles of yin and yang and the life energy Qi; uses traditional formulae and mixtures of herbs, plus other non-drug treatment such as acupuncture (q.v.)

Positive aspects: can be very effective if properly prescribed by herbal practitioner; most common herbs are fairly safe *if quality and purity established*; very fashionable and widely accepted by patients

Negative aspects: lack of regulation; poor quality of some products; toxicity documented for some popular herbs; may interact with conventional drugs; adverse drug reactions possible

The development of TCM and some of its concepts

The study of TCM is a mixture of myth and fact, stretching back well over 5000 years, and TCM still contains many remedies selected for their symbolic significance rather than proven effects (for example, tiger bones to confer strength, ferocity and fearlessness). The herbs are being researched using modern scientific methods and their efficacy is increasingly substantiated.

The discovery of herbal medicine is usually credited to the legendary Chinese Emperor Shen Nong, who ruled around 2800 BC. He is also reputed to have defined the opposing yet complementary principles now known as *yin* and *yang*. Confucius (551–479 BC) established a code of rules and ethics based on the premise that there is an order and harmony of the universe resulting from a delicate balance of yin and yang forces. This philosophy was refined and extended by Dong Zhongshu to include the inner reaches of man himself, i.e. man as the universe on a small scale, containing within himself the locked cycle of yin and yang. Herbal medicine was initially the domain of shamans and mountain recluses, who believed that the mountain mists contained high concentrations of Qi, the vital essence of life. They practised the 'Way of Long Life' which involved diet and herbal medicine, combined with martial arts, a holistic lifestyle that continues today, and in TCM, drugs to rejuvenate and increase longevity are still highly prized.

At this time, herbal medicines were classified into three categories.

- **Upper** – drugs which nurture life
- **Middle** – drugs which provide vitality
- **Lower** – 'poisons' used for serious disease

The most noted physician of these times was Zhang Zhogjing who divided diseases into six types: three 'yin' and three 'yang'. His prescriptions aimed to correct any imbalances of these forces. He also contributed to acupuncture by drawing a map of meridians along which the body's vital energy (Qi) is said to flow. Acupuncture will be dealt with separately in the section on physical therapies (see p.178).

Qi, the essential life force

Qi (pronounced *chi*) permeates everything and is transferable; for example, digestion extracts Qi from food and drink and transfers it to the body while breathing extracts Qi from the air and transfers it to the lungs. These two forms of Qi meet in the blood and form 'human Qi', which circulates through the body. It is the quality, quantity and balance of Qi which determine the state of health and lifespan, and as it is finite, and gradually dissipated throughout life, diet, martial arts, breathing exercises and herbal medicine are used to conserve it.

Yin and yang

The theory of yin and yang still pervades all aspects of Chinese thought. Attributes of both are as follows.

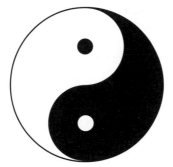

Figure 2.1

- **Yin** – negative, passive, dark, female; associated with water
- **Yang** – positive, active, bright, male; associated with fire

Although the characteristics of the (male) yang appear at first glance to be more exciting and admirable than the (female) yin, in fact yin is considered the stronger. Fire is extinguished by water and water is 'indestructible' and so yin is always put before yang; however, they are always in balance. Consider the well-known symbol in Figure 2.1; where yin becomes weak, yang is strong and vice versa. Both contain the seed of each other, their opposites within themselves. If there is not a proper balance, one may predominate and treatment will be aimed at bringing them back into balance.

The Five Elements and the Vital Organs

These do not correspond to our elements or even our organs exactly, partly because it is the *relationship* between the Vital Organs, the Five Elements, Qi, yin and yang which matters. In addition, exact anatomy was not really understood since until recently, cutting up a

Box 2.2: The Five Elements, linked organs and treatment

Vital Organ	Associated Element
Heart	Fire
Liver	Wood
Spleen	Earth
Lungs	Metal
Kidneys	Water

An illustration of the relationship between the organs and elements, and treatment

The heart is the Vital Organ linked to Fire, and a patient with heart disease or hypertension may have a complexion which is rather red, the colour of fire. This type of person may be a little overweight and enjoy good food and fine wines – the stereotype of the fat and jolly person who laughs a lot, the sound of which is similar to the sound of fire. In TCM this person may be considered to have an over-Fired heart and cooling herbs to 'sedate' the heart will be given, which means reducing blood pressure.

(NB: This is a light-hearted exercise, offering a cartoon picture of a patient, and is in no way intended to insult anyone, offer advice on diagnosis or treatment or cast aspersions on various lifestyles!)

human body (dead or alive) was considered a grave insult to the person, their ancestors and the gods. Each Element is associated with a Vital Organ of the body and will affect the nature of the disease and its treatment, as shown in Box 2.2.

The organs are also considered to be yin or yang and are paired. Coupled organs are connected by meridians, or energy channels, through which Qi flows. Meridians are not associated with the nervous system and cannot be seen physically. They are stimulated with herbs and by acupuncture.

Causes of disease in TCM

If an organ is weak, it may be attacked and therefore should be strengthened. Weakness may be the result of external (cosmological) forces and internal emotional factors. The external forces are called the Six Excesses: Wind, Cold, Summer Heat, Dampness, Dryness and Fire. Most people are not affected by the Six Excesses, unless the body is deficient in Qi or weather conditions are abnormal (i.e. not what is expected for the time of year). The internal factors are the Seven Emotions: joy, anger, anxiety, concentration, grief, fear and fright. Excessive emotional activity causes a severe yin–yang imbalance, blockage of Qi in the meridians and impairment of Vital Organ function. This leads to damage of the organs and allows disease to enter from outside, or a minor weakness from inside to develop. There are a few other causes (e.g. epidemics, insect and animal bites, hereditary diseases) which are not emotional or external excesses but these are the exception, not the rule, and whatever the cause, once actual physical damage has occurred, treatment must be instigated.

Diagnosis may involve any of the following: examination of the tongue, pulse diagnosis (more than one pulse will be taken, depending on the pressure exerted), palpation of internal organs and massage (to detect temperature and knotted muscles or nerves), and interviewing (questions are asked about sleep patterns, tastes in food and drink, stool and urine quality, fever, perspiration and sexual activity). This is the preserve of the TCM practitioner rather than the pharmacist but detailed information can be obtained from books cited in the further reading list.

Treatment in TCM

The purpose is to promote harmony and restore Qi and the yin–yang balance. For example, a fever would be characterized as a hot (yang) disease and would be treated with a cooling (yin) herb, as shown in Table 2.1. It is interesting to note that malaria (a febrile disease) is treated in TCM by sweet wormwood, *Artemisia annua* (a yin herb), and modern research has shown the plant to contain a powerful antiprotozoal compound (artemisinin), which is now in clinical use as an antimalarial, and the source of a semisynthetic anti-malarial, artemether. A disease of Qi deficiency would be treated with a Qi-nourishing herb, e.g. ginseng, as shown.

These are just a couple of examples. Specialist diagnosis and prescribing are the province of the trained TCM practitioner.

Once the prescription has been chosen and written out, the patient takes it to a Chinese herbalist or pharmacist who prepares the remedy. The patient may be given a crude herb mixture with instructions on how to prepare it at home, perhaps as an infusion or tea. Pastes and pills are prepared by the herbalist and may take several days to complete. Slow-release preparations are made using beeswax pills; tonic wines, fermented dough (containing herbs) and external poultices are also common. As far as pharmacists are concerned, there are now preparations available, notably Dong Qai, Astragalus, Dan Shen and Reishi mushroom, which are becoming increasingly well known to the public. These may be purchased from a pharmacy or information may be requested by patients. Their safety profile and drug interactions are given in Table 2.6.

Table 2.1 Treatment of disease in TCM according to the yin and yang nature of the disease and the remedy

Type of disease	Example of disease	Nature of disease	Nature of remedy	Example of remedy	Desired effect
Cold	Nausea, vomiting	Yin	Yang	Ginger (*Zingiber officinale*)	Warming
Hot	Malaria, fever	Yang	Yin	Sweet wormwood (*Artemisia annua*)	Cooling
External, Hot	Psoriasis	Yang	Yin	Burdock (*Arctium lappa*)	Cooling
Empty	Fatigue, diabetes	Qi deficiency	Tonic	Ginseng (*Panax ginseng*)	Nourishing

Ayurveda

Principles: holistic; based on an ancient system of balance and harmony epitomized by the Tridosha (three basic humours or forces) and the life energy, Prana; uses traditional formulae and mixtures of herbs and minerals; has a great emphasis on cleansing the system

Positive aspects: can be very effective if properly prescribed by a practitioner; most common herbs are fairly safe if purity established; very fashionable

Negative aspects: lack of regulation; poor quality of some products; some formulae include toxic metals such as lead and arsenic; safety concerns about some popular herbs; may interact with conventional drugs; adverse drug reactions possible

The development of Ayurveda and some of its concepts

Ayurveda is a system of sacred Hindu medicine which originated in India over 5000 years ago. It now accommodates modern science, especially in relation to the testing of medicines, and research and adaptation are actively encouraged.

In Ayurveda, the patient is unique and is therefore subject to unique imbalances. There is a life force, which can be nourished, protected and, of course dissipated. There are three opposing principles or 'humours', the Tridosha, whose balance is vital to health. Many remedies are common to both Ayurveda and TCM although the philosophical rationale for their application may be a little different. There are only a few Ayurvedic practitioners ('Vaid') in the West at present but its popularity is growing rapidly and Ayurvedic medicines are now being imported to many other countries. Many ethnic populations from India and Pakistan continue to use their own traditional remedies whilst living in

Europe, Australia or the US and philosophically, Ayurveda has similarities with Traditional Chinese Medicine.

Prana, the life energy

Prana activates both body and mind; it is seated in the head and governs emotions, memory, thought and other functions of the mind. Nutrient Prana from the air gives energy to the vital Prana in the brain, via respiration, and is thus equivalent to Qi in Chinese medicine. Prana kindles the bodily fire, Agni, and thus governs the functioning of the heart, entering the bloodstream from which it controls the vital organs (Dhatus).

The five elements (Bhutas)

Ether (space), air, fire, water and earth are the basic elements in Ayurveda; they are manifestations of cosmic energy and related to the five senses of hearing, vision, touch, taste and smell, and therefore to related activity. For example, ether is related to hearing (since sound is transmitted through it) and from there is connected to the ear (the associated sense organ), leading to speech and involving the 'organs of action' which are the tongue and vocal cords. Fire is similarly associated with the eyes (sense organs), leading to actions such as walking, by the organs of action, the feet.

Tridosha: Vata, Pitta and Kapha, the three humours

The five basic elements combine and manifest in the human body as three basic forces or humours known as the Tridosha (Table 2.2). These are known as Vata, Pitta and Kapha (individually called Doshas) and they govern

Table 2.2 *Determining the human constitution according to the Tridosha*

Aspect of constitution	Vata character	Pitta character	Kapha character
Bodyweight	Low	Moderate	Overweight
Skin	Dry, cool, rough	Oily, warm, soft	Oily, cool
Eyes	Small, dark	Sharp, green/grey	Large, blue
Hair	Dark, dry, curly	Fair, oily	Dark or fair, thick, oily
Appetite	Poor or variable	Good or excessive	Healthy, steady
Thirst	Variable	Excessive	Reduced
Mentality	Restless, active	Aggressive, intelligent	Calm, slow
Emotional temperament	Insecure, unpredictable	Irritable, aggressive	Calm, acquisitive
Speech	Fast	Strong	Slow
Physical activity	Active	Moderate	Lethargic
Sleep	Poor, interrupted	Little, sound	Heavy, long

Adapted from Heinrich M, Barnes J, Gibbons S, Williamson EM 2003 Fundamentals of pharmacognosy and phytotherapy. Elsevier, Edinburgh, with permission.

all functions of the body and mind, including basic human emotions such as fear, anger and greed, and more complicated sentiments like empathy and compassion. Diagnosis and treatment of disease require an understanding of the relationship between them (as with yin and yang in TCM). Additionally, some similarities can be drawn with the humoral theory of Western traditional herbal medicine. When the Tridosha is in harmony and functions in a balanced manner, the result is health and a feeling of well-being; however, in cases of imbalance and disharmony, the result is disease.

The characteristics of the Tridosha can be simplified as follows.

- **Vata** – affiliated to air or ether (space); the principle of movement. Associated with the central nervous system and governs breathing, all forms of motion, heartbeat and nervous impulses
- **Pitta** – affiliated to fire and water; governs body temperature and energy. It therefore governs metabolism, endocrine function, digestion and excretion and is concerned with intelligence and understanding
- **Kapha** – associated with water and earth. It is responsible for physical and biological structure, regulation of immunity, production of bodily fluids (mucus, synovial fluid) and assists with wound healing, general vigour and memory retention

The human constitution (Prakruti)

The constitution of an individual (Prakruti) is determined by the state of the parental Tridosha *at conception*. Most people are not completely one type or another but can be described as Vata-Pitta or Pitta-Kapha, for example. Certain characteristics are associated with each type; for example, people of Vata constitution are generally physically underdeveloped with cold, rough, dry and cracked skin. Table 2.3 indicates constitution in a superficial way, but it is not a tool for self-diagnosis. As well as the Vata, Pitta and Kapha types of personality, other attributes also provide the basis for individual differences and dispositions.

The digestive fire (Agni) and the waste products (Ama)

Agni governs metabolism and is essentially Pitta in nature. An imbalance in the Tridosha will impair Agni

56

Table 2.3   Effect of different foods on the Tridosha

Dosha Food type	Vata Aggravates	Balances	Pitta Aggravates	Balances	Kapha Aggravates	Balances
Meat	Lamb, pork, venison	Beef, eggs, chicken, turkey (white meat)	Beef, lamb, pork, egg yolk	Chicken, turkey (all), egg white	Beef, lamb, pork, seafood	Chicken, turkey (dark meat), eggs
Cereals	Rye, barley	Cooked oats, rice, wheat	Brown rice	White rice, wheat, barley	Cooked oats rice, wheat	Barley, rye, maize (corn)
Vegetables	Raw veg, cauliflower, sprouts, peas, cabbage, aubergine, lettuce, mushrooms, onion (raw), potatoes	Cooked veg, carrots, garlic, green beans, cucumber, avocado, courgettes	Carrots, aubergine, garlic, onion, spinach, tomatoes, hot peppers	Broccoli, sprouts, lettuce, peas, cauliflower, mushrooms, courgettes	Cucumber, tomatoes, courgettes	Cauliflower, sprouts, cabbage, carrots, aubergine, lettuce, mushrooms, onions, peas, potatoes
Fruit	Dried fruit, apples, pears, watermelon	Sweet fruits, apricots, peaches, bananas, cherries, grapes, citrus	Sour fruits, peaches, bananas, grapes, lemons, oranges, pineapple	Sweet fruits, apples, melon, coconut, raisins, prunes	Bananas, coconut, grapefruit, grapes, lemon, orange, melon, pineapple	Apples, apricots, peaches, pears, cherries, raisins, prunes

Dairy	All OK	All OK	Buttermilk, cheese, yogurt	Butter, milk	None	Goat's milk
Oils	All OK	All OK	Corn, sesame, almond	Sunflower, soya, olive	None	None
Seasoning	All OK	All OK	Most	Coriander, fennel, turmeric	All	Salt

Adapted from Heinrich M, Barnes J, Gibbons S, Williamson EM 2003 Fundamentals of pharmacognosy and phytotherapy. Elsevier, Edinburgh, with permission.

Notes:

1. Foods which aggravate a particular Dosha should not be taken in excess by a person of that constitution, e.g. a Vata person should not take excessive amounts of lamb, cabbage, potatoes or dried fruits. However, eggs, rice, cooked vegetables and sweet fruits would be beneficial to someone of Vata constitution.

2. The table can also be used to decide which type of food to eat in different seasons, e.g. in summer, Pitta predominates and those foods which aggravate Pitta should be avoided, so seafood, melon and cow's milk products drinks are not recommended then. Autumn is the season of Vata, Spring is Kapha-Pitta.

and food will not be digested or absorbed properly. The three waste products (Ama) are the faeces, urine and sweat; production and elimination of these are vital to health. Their appearance and properties can give many indications of the state of the Tridosha and therefore health. As an example, the colour of urine depends on the diet and if the patient has a fever or jaundice (Pitta disorders), it may be darker. Substances such as coffee and tea, which stimulate urination, also aggravate Pitta and render the urine dark yellow. Overactive Ama is also detrimental, in that overcombustion of nutrients may occur, leading to Vata disorders and emaciation.

The seven tissues (Dhatus) and the attributes (Gunas)

In Ayurveda, the human body consists of seven basic tissues or organs; when there is a disorder in the balance of the Tridosha, the Dhatus are directly affected. Health can be maintained by taking steps to keep Vata-Pitta-Kapha in balance through a proper diet, herbal treatment and exercise programme. The Dhatus do not correspond to our definition of anatomy but are more a tissue type than an individual organ.

Ayurveda also encompasses a subtle concept of attributes or qualities called Gunas, which contain potential energy while their associated actions express kinetic energy. Vata, Pitta and Kapha each have their own attributes, and substances having similar attributes will tend to aggravate the related bodily humour.

Causes of disease in Ayurveda

In Ayurveda, a state of health exists when the Tridosha and the digestive fire (Agni) are in a balanced condition.

When the balance of any of these systems is disturbed, the disease process begins. Diseases and disorders are ascribed to Vata, Pitta and Kapha and are treated with the aid of medicines possessing the opposite attribute, to try to correct the deficiency or excess. The Tridosha has also recently been defined as the equilibrium and co-ordination between the three vital body systems, i.e. the central nervous system (CNS), which corresponds to Vata, the endocrine system to Pitta and the immune axis to Kapha, all operating with positive and negative feedback.

Other analogies with modern science have been attempted, in that the Tridosha can be considered to govern all metabolic activities: catabolism (Vata), metabolism (Pitta) and anabolism (Kapha). When Vata is out of balance, the metabolism will be disturbed, resulting in excess catabolism (the breakdown or deterioration process in the body) and excess Vata would therefore induce emaciation. When anabolism is greater than catabolism (excess Kapha), there is an increased rate of growth and repair of organs and tissues. Excess Pitta disturbs metabolism generally.

Diagnosis involves taking more than just a case history; astrological considerations, as well as karma, the good and bad effects across reincarnations, are also taken into account. This is a complicated system outside the scope of this book; the further reading list contains a number of references which deal with aspects of diagnosis. A thorough medical examination, where the appearance of the tongue, properties of the urine, sweat and sputum are examined, will also be performed.

Treatment

This may involve diets, bloodletting, fasting, skin applications and enemas used to cleanse the system. There is a drastic programme consisting of five types of detoxification, known as Panchkarma, which is used to

Table 2.4 *Effect on the Tridosha of some herbs*

Botanical name	Ayurvedic name	Effect on dosha	Medical use
Aegle marmelos Bengal quince	Bael, Bel	Promotes Pitta	Antidysenteric, digestive, tonic
Andrographis paniculata Green chiretta	Kalmegh	Pacifies Kapha and Pitta	Liver protectant, jaundice
Ocimum sanctum Holy basil	Tulsi	Pacifies Vata and Kapha	Expectorant, febrifuge, immunomodulator
Phyllanthus emblica Indian gooseberry	Amla	Balances Tridosha	Improves memory and intelligence, tonic
Piper nigrum Black pepper	Kalmirch	Pacifies Vata and Pitta	Digestive, respiratory disorders
Swertia chirata Chiretta	Chirayita	Balances Tridosha	Appetite stimulant, liver disorders
Withania somnifera Winter cherry	Ashwagandha	Pacifies Vata and Kapha	Analgesic, sedative, rejuvenator

cleanse the system. Drugs may then be given to bring the Tridosha and the Dhatus into balance again. These include herbal treatments as well as minerals – and there are thousands in use (Table 2.4). In addition, yogic breathing and other techniques are used. Even now, in modern Indian medicine the Ayurvedic properties of medicines may be described, together with conventional therapeutic and phytochemical data. Herbs are prepared as tinctures, pills, powders and some unique formulations.

Ayurveda is very metaphysical, far too much so for many Westerners to grasp, but many of the herbs have a sound basis in pharmacology and can be used without a deep understanding of its philosophy.

Rasayana

Rasayana are essentially panaceas, affecting many systems of the body and producing a tonifying and generally positive effect on health. In general, modern research has found them to have antioxidant, immuno-modulating and various other beneficial activities.

Three well-known ones are *Piper longum* (black pepper), *Phyllanthus emblica* (Indian gooseberry) and *Withania somnifera* (Ashwagandha).

Anthroposophical medicine

Principles: an attempt to describe health and natural medicine in more spiritual terms; considered an adjunct to conventional medicine rather than an alternative

Positive aspects: holistic; generally considered to be safe; widely accepted in Germany where anthroposophical hospitals are well established

Negative aspects: non-scientific, little evidence for some treatments; mistletoe therapy for cancer has given cause for concern (but only if patients refuse conventional chemotherapy)

62

Anthroposophical medicine is a perception of health and disease based on the work of Rudolf Steiner (1861–1925), and uses herbs and minerals, often in combinations. Steiner described how the soul and spirit affect health and considered that there are four manifestations of the body, and three systems by which they can function. Steiner believed that health is maintained when the three systems are in harmony and that disharmony results in illness – a common theme throughout all forms of herbal medicine.

The four body manifestations are:

- the physical body
- the etheric body (life force)
- the astral body (conscious awareness)
- the spiritual body (self-awareness or ego).

The three functional systems are:

- the 'sense-nervous' system (located in the head and spinal column), concerned with 'cooling' and 'hardening' processes, and expressed in terms of diseases such as arthritis

- the 'reproductive-metabolic' system, which includes the parts of the body that are constantly in motion (located mainly in the limbs and digestive system), concerned with 'warming' and 'softening' processes, relevant to conditions such as fevers
- the 'rhythmic' system (located in the heart, lungs and circulation) which connects and balances the other two systems.

Anthroposophic medicines are derived mainly from plants and minerals, such as calcium, iron and copper. The ingredients may be 'potentized', in a similar way to homeopathic preparations (q.v.), but with lower dilutions. Thus, many anthroposophical medicines will still contain measurable amounts of ingredients and can be considered to be herbal medicines.

Modern anthroposophical medicine is still holistic but diagnosis now involves conventional methods, including laboratory investigations, as well as the traditional approach where the lifestyle of the patient, their behaviour and artistic temperament are also considered. Practitioners use a range of therapies, including diet, therapeutic massage and prescribed movements (known as eurythmy) and art therapy, in addition to herbs and minerals. There is a wide range of medicines available for the symptomatic relief of conditions deemed suitable for self-medication, and in Germany, Switzerland and The Netherlands there are specialist hospitals dedicated to anthroposophical medicine.

Mistletoe therapy

One of the most popular and widely used types of anthroposophical medicine is the range of products known as Iscador, which are derived from mistletoe and used in the treatment of cancer. There are several different preparations containing fermented aqueous extracts of mistletoe (*Viscum album*). Since mistletoe is a semiparasite, extracting phytochemicals as well as water and minerals from the host, the constitution differs according to the host plant. The range includes:

- Iscador M: extract of mistletoe grown on apple trees (*Malus* species)
- Iscador P: extract of mistletoe grown on pine trees (*Pinus* species)
- Iscador Qu: extract of mistletoe grown on oak trees (*Quercus* species).

The different mistletoe products are prescribed for patients with different types of cancer. Treatment is usually given by subcutaneous injection, although the intravenous injection route is sometimes used and oral formulations are also available. Mistletoe therapy should be supervised by a qualified practitioner in view of the serious nature of the conditions it is recommended for (i.e. cancer) and because it is usually administered by injection.

COMMENTS ON TRADITIONAL HERBAL MEDICINE SYSTEMS

It is now obvious that the same herbs are often used by several herbal medicine systems, even though the philosophies behind the therapies are different, which gives a good indication as to the reliability of their indications. An example of this is the herb (or spice or food) ginger. According to Grieve (1931), in traditional medical herbalism in the UK, ginger was used for digestive complaints, having been introduced into Europe in the 1500s. Mills & Bone (2000) consider ginger to be an evidence-based medicine, which qualifies as rational phytotherapy. In TCM, ginger is designated a yang (hot) herb and thus is suitable for treating yin (cold) diseases, such as nausea and vomiting. In Ayurveda, the properties of ginger are described as pungent and it is used for diseases characterized by an excess of Kapha (cold, wet) and Vata (cold, dry), which again includes sickness.

Even without any knowledge of the philosophy or principles of these therapies, it is possible to use the remedies advocated, with benefit and without harm, provided that normal precautions are taken with regard to quality, formulation, dose and combination with conventional therapies.

65

CHOOSING A HERBAL OR NUTRACEUTICAL REMEDY

Many patients know what they want before they enter the pharmacy; others have heard of one or more remedies which they are keen to investigate and then try; yet more are distressed at the failure of conventional therapies and are desperate to try anything. In all cases the patient is entitled to expect that the pharmacist will be able to advise; after all, these are still medicines and the pharmacist is *the* expert on medicines, whether in the medical information department of a hospital or in the high street dispensary. Table 2.5 can be used to suggest a remedy and in Table 2.6 you can check details of the individual remedy. This gives more information (where known) as to suitability, dose, safety and possible drug–herb interactions. There are large gaps in our knowledge of some aspects of these products but rather than discouraging their use, it would probably be more practical to ask patients to report back problems to the pharmacist so these can be documented which will help to improve the safety of these natural medicines.

REGULATION OF HERBAL MEDICINES IN THE UK

The regulations pertaining to herbal medicinal products (HMPs) in Europe are very complicated, widely flouted and currently under review, and so will be dealt with briefly. Common legal categories (P, POM), will not be explained as the pharmacist has many sources of references to the regulations.

At present, HMPs are available on the UK market as:

- licensed herbal medicines
- herbal medicines exempt from licensing (under section 12 of the Medicines Act)
- unlicensed herbal products, sold as food or dietary supplements
- pharmacy-only medicines (P)
- prescription-only medicines (POM).

Many problems arise from the fact that most HMPs are not licensed as medicines but are sold as unlicensed products. Lack of legal control has led to herbal safety problems occurring as a result of inadequate (or adulterated or just plain fraudulent) quality.

Licensed herbal medicines and the new THMPD

Most of the existing licensed herbal products in the UK were granted a product licence of right (PLR) because they were already on the market when the Medicines Act was introduced. When these PLRs were reviewed in the 1990s, manufacturers of HMPs which were intended for use *in minor or self-limiting conditions* could rely on bibliographic evidence to support their use, rather than being required to carry out new clinical trials. In other parts of Europe more HMPs are licensed but generally speaking, licensed products are in a minority and the law is not working well, a fact which has led to the introduction of the new regulatory framework for herbal medicines, the Traditional Herbal Medicinal Product Directive (THMPD). This is a European Union (EU) directive which is meant to establish a new, harmonized legislative framework. It constitutes a simplified registration procedure, based on quality and safety, and relying on evidence of traditional use to support efficacy. It is meant to provide some form of public safeguard for controlling traditional HMPs which could not otherwise fulfil medicines licensing criteria.

The main features are that manufacturers must provide:

- evidence that the herb has been used traditionally for more than 30 years (although 15 years' non-EU use will be taken into account – important for Asian HMPs)
- bibliographic data on safety, with an expert report and a quality dossier demonstrating manufacture according to principles of good manufacturing practice (GMP).

The THMPD is not intended as a route to licensing POMs or for traditional herbal medicines that should be licensed by the conventional route. The THMPD will accommodate ethnic medicines that have been used in the UK (or any other member state) for at least 15 years. The directive is in force as from October 2005 but there will be a 5-year transition period for manufacturers to meet requirements.

Unlicensed herbal medicines

HMPs exempt from licensing are those 'compounded and supplied by herbalists on their own recommendation' (as specified under section 12(1) of the Medicines Act 1968), and 'those consisting solely of dried, crushed or comminuted (fragmented) plants'. They must not contain any non-herbal 'active' ingredients and are sold under their botanical name and with no written recommendations for use. These exemptions were intended to give CAM practitioners (herbalists) the flexibility to prepare their own remedies for their patients (even though there is no statutory regulation of herbalists in the UK yet). Herbal medicines that are 'industrially produced' are required to hold a marketing authorization but this term is not defined in law and small-scale manufacturers have been permitted to sell products under the exemption without legal challenge. Many herbal products are marketed as food supplements, without making medical claims, and are regulated under the Food Act of 1990, rather than the Medicines Act.

Traditional medicines used in TCM and Ayurveda are subject to the same legislation as 'Western' herbal medicines. In Europe and the US, there are further restrictions on certain toxic herbal ingredients, including *Aristolochia* species.

References and Further reading

Barnes J, Anderson LA, Phillipson JD 2002 Herbal medicines, 2nd edn. Pharmaceutical Press, London.

Bone K 1996 Clinical applications of Ayurvedic and Chinese herbs. Monographs for the Western practitioner. Phytotherapy Press, Queensland, Australia.

Eldin S, Dunford A 1999 Herbal medicine in primary care. Butterworth-Heinemann, Oxford.

Ernst E (ed) 2001 The desk-top guide to complementary and alternative medicine. Mosby, Edinburgh.

Evans WC 2002 Trease and Evans' pharmacognosy, 15th edn. Baillière Tindall, London.

Fragakis AS 2003 The health professional's guide to popular dietary supplements, 2nd edn. American Dietetic Association, Chicago.

Fulder S 1996 The handbook of alternative and complementary medicine, 3rd edn. Oxford University Press, Oxford.

Grieve M 1931 A modern herbal. Jonathan Cape, London.

Heinrich, H, Barnes J, Gibbons S, Williamson EM 2003 Fundamentals of pharmacognosy and phytotherapy. Churchill Livingstone, Edinburgh.

Kayne SB 2002 Complementary therapies for pharmacists. Pharmaceutical Press, London.

Koh H-L, Teo H, Ng H-L 2003 Pharmacists' patterns of use, knowledge, and attitudes to complementary and alternative medicine. Journal of Alternative and Complementary Medicine 9:51–63.

Lad V 1990 Ayurveda: the science of self-healing. Lotus Press, Wisconsin, USA.

Mason P 2001 Dietary Supplements. Pharmaceutical Press, UK.

Mills SY, Bone K 2000 Principles and practice of phytotherapy. Churchill Livingstone, Edinburgh.

Mills SY, Bone K 2005 The essential guide to herbal safety. Churchill Livingstone, Edinburgh.

Okpako DT 1999 Traditional African medicine: theory and pharmacology explored. Trends in Pharmacological Science 20:482–485.

Rapport L, Lockwood B 2001 Nutraceuticals. Pharmaceutical Press, London.

Sairam TV 2000 Home remedies, vols I, II and III. Penguin, Mumbai, India.

Upton R (ed) (1999–2006) American Herbal Pharmacopoeia Monographs (see individual herbs).

Williamson EM (ed) 2002 Major Herbs of Ayurveda. Elsevier, UK.

Williamson EM (ed) 2002 Major herbs of Ayurveda. The Dabur Foundation. Churchill Livingstone, Edinburgh.

Williamson EM 2003 Potter's Cyclopedia herbal medicines. CW Daniels, Saffron Walden, Essex.

Williamson EM 2005 Interactions between herbal and conventional medicines. Expert Opinion in Drug Safety 4(2): 355–378.

Williamson EM 2005 Interactions between herbal and conventional medicines. Expert Opinion in Drug Safety 4(2):355–378.

69

Table 2.5 *Therapeutic indications treated by herbal medicines and supplements*

	Indication	Herbs used
Gastrointestinal system	Nausea and vomiting	Ginger
	Dyspepsia and ulcers	Acidophilus
		Aloe vera
		Artichoke
		Chamomile
		Liquorice
		Peppermint
	Liver disease or protection	Alpha-lipoic acid
		Andrographis
		Artichoke
		Berberis
		Gentian
		Golden seal
		Milk thistle
		Oregon grape
		Schisandra
		Turmeric
	Constipation	Aloes
		Cascara
		Frangula
		Rhubarb
		Senna
	Appetite stimulation	Gentian
		Wormwood
	Weight control	Boldo
		Chitosan
	General tonics, adaptogens and body-building aids	Acidophilus
		Ashwagandha
		Bee pollen
		L-carnitine
		Creatine
		Ginseng
		Guarana
		Octosanol/policosanol
		Ornithine ketoglutarate
		Rhodiola
		Schisandra
	Irritable bowel syndrome	Artichoke
		Peppermint oil

Cardiovascular system	Heart disease and/or hypertension	Dan Shen
		Garlic
		Hawthorn
	Hypercholesterolaemia	Acidophilus
		L-carnitine
		DHA/EPA (fish oil)
		Flaxseed
		Garlic
		Octosanol/policosanol
		Spirulina
		Turmeric
	Venous insufficiency, haemorrhoids, enhancement of visual acuity	Bilberry
		Butcher's broom
		Ginkgo biloba
		Horse chestnut
		Pycnogenol
	Water retention	Dandelion
Respiratory system	Nasal and sinus congestion	Ma Huang (Ephedra)
		Peppermint oil (menthol)
		Thyme oil (thymol)
		Tolu balsam
	Anti-allergic (hayfever)	Butterbur
	Coughs, colds and influenza	Astragalus
		Balm of Gilead
		Coltsfoot
		Echinacea
		Elderflower
		Marshmallow
		Thyme
		Tolu balsam
		Vervain
		White horehound
Central nervous system	Sedatives and hypnotics	Ashwagandha
		Hops
		Lemon balm
		Lettuce, wild
		Melatonin
		Oats
		Passiflora
		Valerian
		Vervain
	Cognition enhancement	Acetyl carnitine
		Ginkgo biloba
		Ginseng
		Rhodiola
		Rosemary
		Sage

71

	Indication	Herbs used
	Stimulants	Ginseng
		Guarana
		Rhodiola
	Antidepressant	St John's wort
Antiinflammatory	Migraine	Feverfew
	Muscle pain, arthritis, rheumatism, etc.	Bromelain
		Butcher's broom
		Cat's claw
		Chondroitin
		Devil's claw
		DHA/EPA (fish oil)
		Glucosamine
		Golden rod
		Meadowsweet
		Turmeric
		Wild yam
		Willow bark
	For external application (for bruising, sprains, etc.)	Arnica
		Calendula
		Chamomile
		Clove oil (inc. dental)
Infectious diseases	Immune stimulants	Aloe vera
		Andrographis
		Astragalus
		Cat's claw
		Echinacea
	Antiinfectives (taken orally)	Bearberry (UTI)
		Berberis
		Buchu (UTI)
		Cranberry (UTI)
		Elderflower
		Goldenseal
		Oregon grape
		Pelargonium
		Sage
		Thyme
	Antiinfectives (applied topically)	Lemon balm
		Tea tree oil
		Tolu balsam
Endocrine system	Female hormonal	Agnus castus
		Black cohosh
		Black haw
		Cramp bark
		DHEA

		Dong Quai
		Evening primrose oil
		Flaxseed
		Raspberry leaf
		Red clover
		Soya
		Starflower oil
		Wild yam
	Male hormonal	DHEA
		Nettle
		Pumpkin seed
		Pygeum bark
		Saw palmetto
Skin	Wound healing, bruising and soreness (for external application)	Aloe vera
		Arnica
		Calendula
		Chamomile
		Gotu kola (both internal and external)
		Ornithine ketoglutarate
		St John's wort oil
	Eczema	Calendula
		Chamomile
		Evening primrose oil (both internal and external)
		Oats
	Acne (taken internally)	Echinacea
		Red clover
	Acne (external application)	Tea tree oil
Hair	Head lice	Insect flowers
		Larkspur
		Tea tree oil
Antioxidants: for chemoprevention, as general 'tonics' and 'antiageing or anti-neurodegenerative agents		Acidophilus
		Alpha-lipoic acid
		Beta-carotene
		Coenzyme Q10
		Ginseng
		Grapeseed
		Green tea
		Lycopene
		Pycnogenol
		Turmeric

Table 2.6 Common nutritional and herbal supplements: a summary of their uses, doses and interactions with prescription and OTC medicines

Supplement Compound or herb Botanical or dietary source Type of constituents	Clinical use Traditional and modern, evidence, toxicity, side effects and contraindications	Usual dosage ranges Herb, extract equivalent or doses used in clinical trials	Drug interactions Reports and recommendations based on clinical or sound theoretical grounds
Acetyl L-carnitine *Dietary amino acid*	Cognitive enhancement. Evidence inconclusive, but accumulating. Considered safe in recommended doses	1–2 g daily, in divided doses	None known
Acidophilus (*Lactobacillus acidophilus*; LA) Bacteria found in yogurt and 'health drinks' containing live cultures. Advertised as 'friendly bacteria'!	Reduction of blood cholesterol levels; used to recolonize the gut after taking antibiotics and prevent diarrhoea and/or Candida infection; to improve digestion and absorption of nutrients. Some preliminary evidence	10–20 billion viable LA cells daily; about 2 cups live cultured yogurt	No interactions or contraindications known
Agnus castus (chaste tree) *Vitex agnus castus* Powdered fruit (seed) and extract. Diterpenes, e.g. vitexilactone; flavonoids, e.g. casticin; iridoids, e.g. aucubin, agnoside	Used for menstrual disorders and menopause symptoms. Supporting clinical trial evidence.	1:5 tincture: 1–5 ml daily; 500 mg tablets:1–2 daily; however in Germany, lower doses are successfully used: 30–40 mg crushed fruit, once daily	None known. Theoretical possibility of interacting with dopaminergic drugs; avoid concurrent hormone therapy

Aloes *Aloe ferox, A. barbadensis,* etc. Resinous exudate from cut leaf. Anthraquinone (AQ) glycosides, e.g. aloinosides, free aloe-emodin	Well-proven stimulant laxative. Should not be taken for long periods (see Senna). Some toxicity concerns. Avoid in obstructive bowel disorders	Powdered resin: 100–300 mg when required for *occasional* constipation. Tincture BPC 1949: 2–8 ml	None reported. Avoid regular use with thiazide diuretics and corticosteroids to prevent electrolyte imbalance
Aloe vera Gel or juice extracted from centre of the fleshy leaves of *Aloe* plants (see above) Lectins (aloctins); polysaccharides (acemannan); enzymes, e.g carboxypeptidases	Applied externally to burns and wounds, taken internally as a general tonic, to boost immune system in HIV (acemannan is immune enhancing and antiviral in vitro) and calm GI symptoms	Variable. For internal use, in absence of safety data, not more than 1.2 L day recommended. Acemannan use in HIV from 800–1600 mg (corresponds to 0.5–1 L juice)	None known
Alpha–lipoic acid (ALA, thioctic acid) 1,2-dithiolane-3-pentanoic acid, a dietary antioxidant found in yeast and liver	Antioxidant, especially for use in neurodegenerative diseases (inc. multiple sclerosis and diabetic neuropathy); enhancement of athletic performance; liver protection. Formerly used for liver disease and mushroom (*Amanita* species) poisoning. Some inconclusive evidence	100–800 mg daily, sometimes higher. Well tolerated in doses up to 2000 mg daily	Contraindicated in thiamine deficiency, e.g. in alcoholics, unless given with thiamine supplementation. No others known

Supplement Compound or herb Botanical or dietary source Type of constituents	Clinical use Traditional and modern, evidence, toxicity, side effects and contraindications	Usual dosage ranges Herb, extract equivalent or doses used in clinical trials	Drug interactions Reports and recommendations based on clinical or sound theoretical grounds
Arnica *Arnica montana* Extract of flowers Sesquiterpene lactones, e.g. helenalin, arnifolin, arnicolides; flavonoids, e.g. eupafolin, hispidulin; essential oil, e.g. thymol	Used externally to treat bruising and muscle pain. Immunostimulant. Should not be taken internally (except at homeopathic doses)	Arnica Flower Tincture BPC (for external use, apply three times daily) Arnica cream: for concentration and directions see manufacturers' instructions	None known
Artichoke (globe artichoke) *Cynara scolymus* Extract of leaf. Sesquiterpene lactones, e.g cynaropicrin; phytosterols, e.g taraxasterol; flavonoids and caffeic acid derivatives	Digestive, liver protectant. Used for IBS (irritable bowel syndrome) with supporting clinical trial evidence, and for dyspepsia and hypercholesterolaemia	Herb: 6 g daily in divided doses Standardized extract (as tablets): up to 2 g daily. Taken with meals	None known

Ashwagandha
Withania somnifera
Extract of root
Steroidal lactones, e.g. withanolides, withaferin withasomniferols; alkaloids, e.g. cuscohygrine, ashwagandhine; phytosterols, e.g. sitoindosides

Sedative, tonic, antiinflammatory. Important Ayurvedic herb with some supporting clinical trial evidence

3–6 g powdered root or equivalent extract daily

Potentiates sedative effects of barbiturates and some benzodiazepines; avoid with other sedatives as a precaution

Astragalus
Astragalus membranaceus
Extract of root
Triterpene saponins, e.g. astragalosides, agroastragalosides, astramembranins; isoflavones, e.g. formononetin; polysaccharides, e.g. astragaloglucans

Immune stimulant, tonic. Important Chinese herb with some supporting clinical trial evidence. Used in TCM in a similar way to echinacea (q.v.) in the West

10–30 g dried root per day as decoction (higher doses used by TCM practitioners) 1:2 liquid extract: 4–8 ml

Potentiates activity of aciclovir and some interleukins in animals. Avoid with immunosuppressive agents as a precaution

Balm of Gilead (poplar buds)
Populus spp.
Extract of sticky buds collected in spring before opening. Phenolic glycosides, e.g. populin, salicin; essential oil, e.g. bisabolene, caryophyllene, cineole

Respiratory stimulant and expectorant: used in cough medicines; antiseptic: applied externally in ointment base for inflammation, rheumatism and skin diseases. Little clinical evidence but long history of traditional use

Dried leaf buds 4 g three time daily as an infusion, or equivalent extract

No clinical reports, but for internal use, as it contains salicylates, avoid with other NSAIDs, warfarin, methotrexate, phenytoin, valproate, spironolactone as a precaution

Supplement Compound or herb Botanical or dietary source Type of constituents	Clinical use Traditional and modern, evidence, toxicity, side effects and contraindications	Usual dosage ranges Herb, extract equivalent or doses used in clinical trials	Drug interactions Reports and recommendations based on clinical or sound theoretical grounds
Bearberry (uva-ursi) *Arctostaphylos uva-ursi* Extract of leaf. Hydroquinones, e.g. arbutin, methylarbitun; iridoids, polyphenolic acids and flavonoids	Urinary antiseptic. Usually used in combination products. Excessive use may irritate kidney	1.5–4 g dried leaf or equivalent extract three times daily; preparations (tablets, liquid extract) containing 400–840 mg arbutin daily in divided doses. Not for prolonged internal use	None known. Requires urine to be alkaline for any effect, so avoid with agents causing urine acidity (e.g. ammonium chloride, ascorbic acid)
Bee pollen Powdered pollen collected by bees, mixed with bee secretions, obtained from hives. Protein, trace minerals and vitamins	Source of nutrients, vitamins and minerals; used as a general tonic. No supporting evidence as yet	Powdered bee pollen 3–7 g daily; some recommend capsules of 500 mg taken three times daily	Anaphylaxis reported in some subjects with allergies to bee stings. Avoid in these cases
Berberis (barberry) *Berberis vulgaris* and other spp. Isoquinoline alkaloids, e.g. berberine, berbamine	Antibacterial, antiprotozoal, antidiarrhoeal, digestive, liver protectant. Berberine alone has been used as an antidiarrhoeal and anti-protozoal	1.5–3 g daily dried root or stem bark; 3–6 ml 1:2 liquid extract; 7–14 ml 1:5 tincture. Higher doses used by practitioners, in acute conditions	None known. Berberine inhibits CYP2D6 and CYP3A4 in vitro

Beta-carotene Carotenoid orange-red pigment found in fruit and vegetables	Antioxidant, chemoprotectant. Epidemiological studies confirm lower cancer risk for high beta-carotene diet but NOT for supplementation with isolated compound	20–50 mg daily; has been used up to 300 mg daily (not recommended)	None known. A precursor of vitamin A so avoid overdosing and in pregnant women
Bilberry (blueberry) *Vaccinium myrtillus* Fresh or dried fruit Anthocyanins, polyphenolic acids and catechins	Peripheral vascular disorders, including venous insufficiency, haemorrhoids, etc. in pregnancy; improvement of visual acuity	20–50 g fresh berries daily (but unrestricted as a food); 1:1 liquid extract 3–6 ml or tablets containing equivalent to 50–120 mg anthocyanins, daily	Considered safe in pregnancy
Black cohosh *Actaea racemosa (Cimicifuga racemosa)* Total herb extract. Triterpene glycosides, e.g. actein, cimicifugosides, racemoside. Presence of isoflavones disputed	Menopausal symptoms. Some supporting clinical trial evidence. No oestrogenic effects reported but some authorities recommend avoidance in breast cancer	Traditional use: 0.5–1 g dried root/rhizome 3–4 times daily; 6–12 ml 1:10 tincture daily. Modern use: extract equivalent to 200 mg day. German Commission E recommends up to 6 months treatment	None known. An unconfirmed report suggested interaction with levothyroxine (hyperthyroidism), but with concurrent administration of irbesartan and alprazolam. Avoid with HRT as a precaution

80

Supplement Compound or herb Botanical or dietary source Type of constituents	Clinical use Traditional and modern, evidence, toxicity, side effects and contraindications	Usual dosage ranges Herb, extract equivalent or doses used in clinical trials	Drug interactions Reports and recommendations based on clinical or sound theoretical grounds
Black haw *Viburnum prunifolium* Extract of bark. Iridoid glycosides, e.g. patrinoside, dihydropenstemoside derivatives	Dysmenorrhoea, uterine tonic. No clinical trial evidence but long history of use	2.5–5 g dried bark as a decoction, three times daily	None known
Boldo *Peumus boldo* Leaf extract. Isoquinoline alkaloids, e.g. boldine, isoboldine	Slimming aid. No clinical trial evidence but long history of use	60–200 mg dried leaf three times daily; higher doses, 2–5 g, have been taken as a tea	None known. Possible interaction with warfarin unproven
Bromelain (pineapple enzymes) *Ananas comosus* Proteolytic enzymes extracted from fruit and stem	Analgesic in arthritic conditions and for 'joint health', antiinflammatory, wound healing. Clinical evidence to support use exists, and is increasing	Usual dose 160–2000 mg daily	None known. May increase blood levels of antibiotics (e.g. tetracycline) if given concurrently

Buchu
Agathosma betulina
Flavonoids, e.g. diosmin, rutin; essential oil, e.g. diosphenol, pulegone, menthone

Diuretic, urinary antiseptic, used mainly for cystitis, etc. Little supportive evidence at present. Avoid large or prolonged doses as may cause renal toxicity

1–2 g leaf, as a tea; tincture 1–5 in 60% alcohol 2–4 ml

None known

Butcher's broom
Ruscus aculeatus
Extract of rhizome or whole plant. Saponin glycosides, e.g. ruscine, ruscoside, aculeosides A and B, based on ruscogenins and neoruscogenins; flavonoids, e.g. rutin

Venous insufficiency, in cases of haemorrhoids, varicose veins, retinopathy, etc. may be taken orally or applied topically. Antiinflammatory for bruising, etc.

Powdered rhizome 1–2 g three times a day; extract 250–500 mg daily (or equivalent to 7–11 mg sapnins, calculated as ruscogenin); ointments and suppositories used for external and rectal administration

None known

Butterbur
Petasites vulgaris
Special extract of herb, root. Sesquiterpene lactones, e.g. petasins, isopetasins, and petasinolides

Antiallergic, especially in seasonal allergic rhinitis, antiinflammatory. Products must not contain toxic pyrrolizidine alkaloids, so fresh untreated plant material should not be used

Dried root: 4–7 g daily. Only purified extracts should be used as per manufacturer's specifications, as these have been treated to remove toxic alkaloids

None known

81

Supplement Compound or herb Botanical or dietary source Type of constituents	Clinical use Traditional and modern, evidence, toxicity, side effects and contraindications	Usual dosage ranges Herb, extract equivalent or doses used in clinical trials	Drug interactions Reports and recommendations based on clinical or sound theoretical grounds
Calendula (marigold) *Calendula officinalis* Infusion of petals or flowerheads (tea), extract, ointment. Triterpenes and saponins, e.g. calendulosides, calendulasaponins, heliantrols, faradol; sesquiterpenes, e.g. officinosides, lolioside; flavonoids, etc.	Antiinflammatory, spasmolytic. Used internally for gastrointestinal disorders, but mainly externally as an ointment for wounds, burns, scalds, nappy rash in babies and sore nipples in breast-feeding women	Flower heads 1–4 g three times a day as an infusion. Ointment containing 10% of an extract as a soothing and healing agent	None known
L-Carnitine (3-hydroxy-4-N-trimethylaminobutyric acid). Dietary amino acid found in high concentrations in heart muscle	Only the L-isomer is biologically active, but the D-isomer is a competitive inhibitor and toxic. L-carnitine used for athletic enhancement, heart disease and in kidney dialysis patients. Few side effects but diarrhoea reported; also fishy urine and body odour. Occasional agitation	Usually 500 mg–1 g daily	None known. Carnitine levels reduced in some patients on valproate, carbamazepine and phenytoin, isotretinoin and pivampicillin but this is an indication for supplementation with carnitine, not avoidance. Avoid products containing racemic mixture of DL-carnitine

83

Cascara *Rhamnus purshianus* Bark. Anthraquinone (AQ) glycosides, e.g. cascarosides, palmidins	Well-known stimulant anthraquinone laxative, use now largely obsolete. Should not be taken for long periods (see Senna). May cause griping. Avoid in obstructive bowel disorders	Powdered bark 1–2.5 g; dry extract 100–300 mg; tablets 1–2 at night, for occasional use only	None reported. Avoid regular use with thiazide diuretics and corticosteroids to prevent electrolyte imbalance
Cat's claw (Uña de gato) *Uncaria tomentosa, U.guianensis* Extract of root, bark, leaves. Oxindole alkaloids, e.g. uncarines, mitraphylline, rhynchophylline	Immune stimulant, antiinflammatory, reputed antitumour effect. Products available often of very poor quality. Wide folk use as anticancer therapy with little positive clinical evidence to date	Powdered herb 0.5–5 g daily; extract 25–300 mg daily	Extracts inhibit CYP3A4 and 2C9, so caution with drugs which are substrates of CYP3A4 (e.g. cancer chemotherapy) and warfarin
Chamomile (German or Hungarian) *Matricaria recutita* **Chamomile (English or Roman)** *Chamaemelum nobile* Infusion of flowers (tea), extract, ointment.	Sedative, antiinflammatory, carminative. Important and popular herbs in Europe and USA with much anecdotal but little clinical evidence. Generally regarded as safe.	Powdered flowers 2–8 g, as infusion; liquid extract 1:1, 2–4 ml Ointment containing 10% of an extract standardized to bisabolol	None known. Extract of Matricaria showed weak inhibition of CYP3A5 in vitro

84

Supplement Compound or herb Botanical or dietary source Type of constituents	Clinical use Traditional and modern, evidence, toxicity, side effects and contraindications	Usual dosage ranges Herb, extract equivalent or doses used in clinical trials	Drug interactions Reports and recommendations based on clinical or sound theoretical grounds
Essential oil, e.g. bisabolol and chamazulene (German); tiglic and angelic acid esters and chamazulene (English); flavonoids, e.g. apigenin, rutin, in both	Frequently applied topically in the form of an ointment as an antiinflammatory, for burns, scalds, nappy rash in babies and especially to nipples in breast-feeding women. Infusion used cosmetically to enhance blonde hair		
Chitosan An aminopolysaccharide (similar to cellulose but containing amino groups) forming the exoskeleton of insects and crustaceans, and found in filamentous fungi. Usually extracted from shellfish	Used as a 'fat buster', 'fat trap' or 'fat magnet' because it binds to lipids in vitro and this has been extrapolated to include binding in the stomach. Some clinical evidence but only when taken in a fat-restricted diet	Usually 500 mg, in the form of capsules, three times daily, with meals	Contraindicated in patients allergic to shellfish, and those with malabsorption syndromes as it may reduce absorbence of fat-soluble vitamins (e.g. A and D). Appears generally safe in moderation, but no long-term safety studies carried out

Chondroitin A glycosaminoglycan (GAG) found in cartilage. Commercial supplements derived from bovine cartilage so unsuitable for vegetarians	Often presented in combination with glucosamine (q.v.). The most abundant GAG in cartilage. Used for arthritis and degenerative diseases of joints and sports injury, with some clinical evidence. Requires long-term treatment	Usual dose 1200 mg daily in divided doses	Safety profile good. Unsuitable for vegetarians on ethical grounds. No other contraindications known, no serious ADRs reported, no interactions and well tolerated, but no long-term studies carried out
Cinchona bark (Jesuit's bark) *Cinchona* species Extract of bark. Quinoline alkaloids, e.g. quinine, quinidine	Bitter tonic, used in 'tonic water' and as source of quinine, an antimalarial drug. Quinine used as prevention for night cramp	Powdered bark, 0.3–1 g; dose equivalent of quinine approximately 300 mg	Quinine alkaloid inhibits CYP2D6 but low levels (as in tonic preparations) have no effect
Cloves *Syzygium aromaticum, (Eugenia caryophyllata)* Essential oil, extract of flower bud. Phenylpropanoids, e.g. eugenol, acetyl eugenol, caryophyllene (in oil) plus tannins, chromones, etc. in bud	Oil used as a local anaesthetic for toothache and mouth ulcers. Stimulant. Oil inhibits some CYP enzymes in vitro. Should not be ingested in large quantities	Clove Oil BP (internal): 0.05–0.2 ml Powdered cloves: 120–300 mg, occasional use only	None reported. None expected when applied externally

Supplement Compound or herb Botanical or dietary source Type of constituents	Clinical use Traditional and modern, evidence, toxicity, side effects and contraindications	Usual dosage ranges Herb, extract equivalent or doses used in clinical trials	Drug interactions Reports and recommendations based on clinical or sound theoretical grounds
Coenzyme Q-10 An electron and proton carrier supporting ATP synthesis. Occurs especially in heart, liver, kidney and pancreas; declines with age	Antioxidant used to treat cardiovascular disease and neurodegeneration. Theoretical evidence provided by age decreasing levels; some preliminary clinical evidence	Usual dose 100–200 mg daily; has been used to 800 mg. Suggested monitoring of renal function if over 600 mg/day over a longer (unspecified) period of time	Well tolerated, some mild gastrointestinal disturbance. No interactions known
Coltsfoot Tussilago farfara Extract of flowers, leaves and root. Mucilage, of acidic polysaccharides, flavonoids, e.g. rutin, hyperoside. Pyrrolizidine alkaloids present in variable amounts; should be absent	Expectorant and demulcent, used in coughs, asthma, laryngitis. Products must not contain toxic pyrrolizidine alkaloids, so fresh untreated plant material should not be used	Powdered herb or root: 0.6–2 g three times daily, or equivalent extract. Only purified extracts should be used, as per manufacturer's specifications, as these have been treated to remove toxic alkaloids	None known
Cramp bark Viburnum opulus Extract of bark. Hydroquinones, e.g. arbutin, methylarbutin; coumarins, e.g. scopoletin; triterpenes, e.g. oleanolic acid; catechins	Spasmolytic in menstrual cramp and leg cramp, and (by herbalists only) to prevent miscarriage	Powdered bark, 2–4 g, as a decoction	None reported

Cranberry *Vaccinium macrocarpon, V. oxycoccus* Juice or freeze-dried juice. Polyphenolic acids, anthocyanins and catechins	Urinary tract infection, e.g. cystitis; especially in long-term low-level infection, and prevention of reoccurrence in susceptible patients	Juice, up to 1 L daily Extract, 400–2000 mg daily	Cases of interaction with warfarin reported; avoid concurrent use
Creatine A peptide found in skeletal muscle, formed from glycine, arginine and methionine. Negligible amounts found in plants	Used to increase strength and stamina in body building, athletics and other sports; in the elderly and in muscular wasting diseases. Some evidence for efficacy. Vegetarians have lower body stores and absorb more from supplements	Maximum 2–5 g/day recommended	Unsuitable for use in renal disease; with water retention and with nephrotoxic drugs (including NSAIDs, ACE inhibitors and cyclosporin). Thought to be ineffective with caffeine
Dan Shen *Salvia miltiorrhiza* Extract of root. Diterpenes, e.g. tanshinone derivatives; polyphenolics, e.g. salvianolic acids, and lithospermic acid B derivatives	Cardiovascular disease, hypertension. Important Chinese herb with some supporting clinical trial evidence. In view of indications, probably not suitable for self-medication	Variable, often found as compound formulation. Usual dose 2 g dried root daily, as equivalent extract	Mixture containing Dan Shen interacts with warfarin. Caution with digoxin. Tanshinone IIA inhibits CYP1A in C57BL/6J but not in DBA/2J mice. Extract inhibited CYPs 1A1/2, 2B1/2, and 2E1 in vitro

Supplement Compound or herb Botanical or dietary source Type of constituents	Clinical use Traditional and modern, evidence, toxicity, side effects and contraindications	Usual dosage ranges Herb, extract equivalent or doses used in clinical trials	Drug interactions Reports and recommendations based on clinical or sound theoretical grounds
Dandelion *Taraxacum officinale* Extract of root or leaf. Sesquiterpene lactones, e.g. taraxacoside; triterpenes, e.g. taraxasterol; taraxol; caffeic acid derivatives	Antiinflammatory, antirheumatic, mild diuretic (folklore use shown by French name: 'pis-en-lit'). No clinical trial evidence but long history of use	Dried leaf: 4–10 g, as a tea Dried root, 2–8 g, as a decoction	None reported. Diuretic effect probably too weak to pose problems
Devil's claw *Harpagophytum procumbens* Root and tuber extract. Iridoids, e.g. harpagide, harpagoside, procumbide	Antiinflammatory. Some supporting clinical trial evidence. Long-term use thought to be safe	3–6 g dried tuber daily; 5:1 extract, 600–1200 mg daily	None known

DHA and EPA (docosahexaenoic acid, eicosapentaenoic acid) Omega-3-fatty acids; found abundantly in fish oils	Taken usually in the form of fish oil (e.g. cod liver, halibut liver, salmon) to reduce atherosclerosis and improve cardiovascular health. Also used as an antinflammatory for arthritis and joint mobility. Supporting epidemiological and clinical evidence	Typical doses (suggested by manufacturers) range: 1–10 g fish oil per day	None known. Theoretically, may enhance effect of anticoagulant drugs, but no increase in bleeding time noted in patients undergoing heart surgery who had been taking 4.3 g daily
DHEA (dehydroepiandrosterone) A hormone precursor of androgens and oestrogens; secreted by the adrenal gland; levels decline with age	Advertised as an antiageing hormone and for androgen and oestrogen deficiency. Increases levels of some hormones, e.g. testosterone, and has oestrogenic activity. Some (not all) clinical trial data positive	25–400 mg or more daily	None known. May elevate blood levels of hormones taken concurrently

Supplement Compound or herb Botanical or dietary source Type of constituents	Clinical use Traditional and modern, evidence, toxicity, side effects and contraindications	Usual dosage ranges Herb, extract equivalent or doses used in clinical trials	Drug interactions Reports and recommendations based on clinical or sound theoretical grounds
Dong Quai (Dang Gui, Chinese angelica) *Angelica sinensis* Root extract. Phthalates, e.g. ligustilide, angelicide; coumarins, e.g. bergapten; essential oil, e.g. carvacrol, isosafrole	Premenstrual syndrome, dysmenorrhoea, endometriosis, menopausal symptoms, anaemia. Important Chinese herb with some supporting clinical trial evidence	Dried root, usually up to 4 g daily (but has been used at 15 g), as a decoction. Liquid extract 1:2, 4–8 ml daily	Possible interaction with warfarin in 1 case; pro-thrombin time lowered with concurrent administration in rabbits. Avoid with cancer chemotherapy as a precaution
Echinacea (coneflower) *Echinacea purpurea* (purple coneflower) *E. pallida* (pale coneflower) *E. angustifolia* (narrow-leaf coneflower) Extract of herb, root and expressed juice. Isobutylamides (not in *E. pallida*); caffeic acid derivatives, e.g. echinacoside (not in *E. purpurea*),	Immune stimulant used especially for URTI, colds and flu. Important and popular herb in Europe and USA with much anecdotal but highly conflicting clinical evidence. Products highly variable in composition and quality. It is usually suggested that Echinacea is taken for a fixed	Generally, commercial products used so follow manufacturer's instructions. *Echinacea pallida* and *E. angustifolia*, dried root, 1.5–4.5 g daily; *E. purpurea:* dried root, 1.5–4.5 g daily; dried herb: 2.5–6 g daily; or equivalent extract. Fresh expressed juice 8–9 ml daily; tincture 1:1 made from	No clinical reports. *E. purpurea* selectively modulates CYP3A enzymes in vitro, reduces oral clearance of substrates of CYP1A2 (not CYP2C9 or CYP2D6). Caution with substrates of CYP3A4 and CYP1A2 (cancer chemotherapy, phenytoin, warfarin, clozapine, theophylline, midazolam) until further evidence available.

cichoric acid (only in *E. purpurea*) and cynarin (only in *E. angustifolia*); polyacetylenes, polysaccharides (in *E. purpurea* herb)	period of time rather than continuously	fresh plant, 3–5 ml daily. These may be increased for short-term use	However, Echinacea species differ chemically so results may not be applicable to all
Elderflower; elderberry *Sambucus nigra* Fluid extract of flower and/or berry. Triterpenes, e.g. ursolic, oleanolic acids; flavonoids and polyphenolics	Colds and influenza. Little clinical trial evidence but long history of use. Safe; used to make drinks including cordials and wine	Dried flowers: 2–4 g three times daily, as herbal tea or extract. Berries: 1:1 extract 0.5 ml three times daily or more	None known
Evening primrose *Oenothera biennis* Oil expressed from seed; major active gamma-linolenic acid (GLA) approx 9%	PMS (premenstrual syndrome), atopic eczema. Evidence for efficacy equivocal	Usually 2–4 g daily, occasionally up to 6 g in eczema	GLA moderately inhibits in vitro activity of CYP3A4, CYP1A2, CYP2C9, CYP2D6 and CYP2C19, but these fatty acids are common in foods. Possible clinical interaction with phenothiazines reported
Feverfew *Tanacetum parthenium* Fresh herb; extract of dried herb. Sesquiterpene lactones, e.g. partholide, santamarine, artemorin; volatile oil	Antiinflammatory; migraine prophylaxis. Some clinical trial evidence but products not equivalent. Long history of use. Fresh leaves used but very bitter tasting	Fresh leaves: 2–3 daily for migraine prophylaxis. Freeze-dried leaf: 50 mg daily; tablet containing 150 mg dried leaf standardized to 0.6 mg parthenolide: 1–2 daily	None reported. Theoretical interaction with antiplatelet drugs postulated, but no changes in blood parameters seen in patients; caution with aspirin

92

Supplement Compound or herb Botanical or dietary source Type of constituents	Clinical use Traditional and modern, evidence, toxicity, side effects and contraindications	Usual dosage ranges Herb, extract equivalent or doses used in clinical trials	Drug interactions Reports and recommendations based on clinical or sound theoretical grounds
Flaxseed (linseed) *Linum usitatissiumum* Seed flower, containing lignans, e.g. secoisolariciresinol and its diglucoside; alpha-linoleic acid (ALA) and linolenic acid (expressed seed oil contains around 50% ALA) cyanogenetic glucosides, e.g. linamarin	Emollient, demulcent. Chemoprotectant for cancer and cardiovascular disease. Powdered seed ('flour') is a food and phyto-oestrogen, used in breads, etc. for reducing menopausal symptoms. Seed oil and flour used for hypercholesterolaemia, systemic lupus erythematosus and other immune disorders. Some epidemiological evidence	Oil: usually 2–9 g daily, but high doses, up to 20 g, have been used, equivalent to 12 g ALA. Flour: up to 50 g daily (also equivalent to 12 g ALA)	No interactions known. Some diarrhoea reported, and prolongation of bleeding time suggests caution if taken with warfarin. Avoid in large amounts during pregnancy due to lack of safety data
Frangula (alder buckthorn) *Rhamnus frangula* Bark. Anthraquinone (AQ) glycosides, e.g. frangulosides, glucofrangulins, palmidins; naphthoquinones	Stimulant AQ laxative. Should not be taken for long periods (see Senna). May cause griping. Avoid in obstructive bowel disorders. Often used combined with bulk laxative, e.g. Sterculia, in products such as Normacol Plus™	Powdered bark, 0.5–2.5 g, or as standardized extract	None reported. Avoid regular use with thiazide diuretics and corticosteroids to prevent electrolyte imbalance

Garlic	Antihypercholesterolaemic,	Dried or fresh bulb, 2–4 g;	Reduction of CYP2E1 activity in
Allium sativum	antiplatelet, antibiotic,	oil up to 12 mg; but very	humans and some animal
Oil, and fresh, dried and/or powdered	antioxidant, expectorant.	variable and mainly	species; no increase in
bulb, sometimes aged or fermented.	Widespread global use in	unrestricted	CYP2B1/2 in humans. Mild
Sulphur-containing compounds, e.g.	foods. Many in vitro, in vivo,		inhibition of P-gp in vitro.
allicin, ajoene, diallyldisulphide,	epidemiological and clinical		Single reports of increased
allylmethyltrisulphide and many	studies to support use;		bleeding time with lisinopril,
more; glycosides, e.g. sativoside,	generally regarded as safe		warfarin, chlorzoxazone.
sulphur-containing peptides,			Reduces bio-availability of the
monoterpenes, etc.			protease inhibitor saquinavir
			and to a lesser extent ritonavir.
			Appears safe with most drugs
			except possibly saquinavir
Gentian	Bitter digestive stimulant,	Powdered root, 0.5–2 g as	None known
Gentiana lutea	tonic, liver protector.	extract. Alkaline Gentian	
Root and rhizome extract.	Stimulates saliva production	Mixture BPC, Acid Gentian	
Iridoids, e.g. gentiopicroside and	and bile flow. Used for poor	Mixture BPC: dose 10–20 m	
amarogentin; xanthones, e.g.	appetite, flatulence and bloating.	before meals	
gentisin; alkaloids, e.g. gentianine;	Long history of use but little		
caffeic acid derivatives	clinical evidence available		

Supplement Compound or herb Botanical or dietary source Type of constituents	Clinical use Traditional and modern, evidence, toxicity, side effects and contraindications	Usual dosage ranges Herb, extract equivalent or doses used in clinical trials	Drug interactions Reports and recommendations based on clinical or sound theoretical grounds
Ginger *Zingiber officinalis* Fresh and dried rhizome, extracts. Pungent principles (phenolics with >C-7 side chains); gingerols (in fresh ginger), shogaols (in dried ginger); essential oil, e.g. zingiberene, bisabolene, zingiberol and many more	Antiemetic, carminative, antiinflammatory. Supporting clinical trial evidence. Popular flavouring in Oriental cooking and confectionary. In TCM fresh ginger is preferred for colds, flu and vomiting, dried ginger for nausea and vomiting, poor appetite and digestion. Considered suitable for morning sickness in pregnancy (up to 2 g daily) but safety not proven conclusively	Fresh root equivalent 500 mg–1 g three times a day; dried root 500 mg three times a day; tablets 500 mg twice to four times daily, tincture 1:5, up to 5 ml daily	None known
Ginkgo *Ginkgo biloba* Leaf extract. Fruit eaten in China. Terpene lactones ginkgolides, bilobalide; flavones ginkgetin,	Very popular worldwide, for improving blood flow to enhance memory and cognition in dementia and for intermittent claudication, with	4–8 g leaf. Most products contain standardized extract; daily dose usually 120 mg containing about 30 mg flavones and 10 mg terpene lactones	Most reports unconfirmed. No effect on CYP1A2, CYP3A4, CYP 2E1 CYP2D6 activity in humans, but moderate inducer of CYP2C19. Interaction reported

isoginkgetin bilobetin; ginkgolic acids (in small amounts; more present in fruits)	some supporting clinical trial evidence. May require long-term usage (>6 weeks) before effect seen. Sold also for erectile dysfunction (without evidence). Ginkgolic acids suspected of causing allergies (but no clinical evidence)	(twice this dose has been used in some trials)	with omeprazole in Chinese patients. INRs should be monitored with warfarin, and caution if taken with antiplatelet drugs (aspirin), alprazolam, donezepil and trazodone. Avoid with anticancer drugs
Ginseng (Korean, red) *Panax ginseng* Root extract, often roasted and fermented **American ginseng** *Panax quinquefolius* Other species used include *Panax notoginseng* and *P. pseudoginseng*. **Siberian ginseng** *Eleutherococcus senticosus* Triterpene saponins, in *Panax* these are ginsenosides, e.g. ginsenoside Rg1 (major) and notoginsenosides; in *Eleutherococcus* eleutherosides A–F. *Panax* contains polysaccharides, e.g. panaxans A–F, and polyacetylenes, e.g. panaxydol	Chinese herb now very popular worldwide. An 'adaptogen' used to improve physical and mental stamina and enhance virility. Supporting clinical trial evidence. Usually taken for courses of up to 3 months; longer term appropriate in the elderly or chronically unwell. Considered safe, although some evidence of oestrogenic effects or overstimulation at very high doses	Use in the West, dried root 0.5–3 g daily. TCM practitioners use higher doses, 1–10 g dried root, or up to 30 g in cases of shock, usually as a decoction. 1:2 liquid extract: 1–6 ml daily. 5:1 standardized extract, 200 mg daily	Suspected potentiation of phenelzine and nifedipine (a CYP3A4 substrate) in animal study. Varied enzyme-selective effects on other CYPs depending on nature of extract. Ginsenosides inhibit P-gp moderately at high concentrations. Avoid with MAOIs, nifedipine, and in cancer chemotherapy. American ginseng (*P. quinquefolius*) reduced effects of warfarin in healthy volunteers, but *Panax ginseng* had no effect

Supplement Compound or herb Botanical or dietary source Type of constituents	Clinical use Traditional and modern, evidence, toxicity, side effects and contraindications	Usual dosage ranges Herb, extract equivalent or doses used in clinical trials	Drug interactions Reports and recommendations based on clinical or sound theoretical grounds
Glucosamine An amino-monosaccharide composed of glutamic acid and glucose, found in connective tissue	Precursor of glycosaminoglycan (GAG), a component of cartilage, which is synthesized by the body, an ability which decreases with age. Widely used for arthritis and degenerative diseases of joints, with clinical evidence. Requires long-term treatment	1.5 g in daily divided doses, can be decreased to 1 g (as maintenance dose) when improvement seen	Safety profile good. No interactions reported. Occasional diarrhoea and GI side effects avoided by taking with food
Golden rod *Solidago virgaurea* Extract of leaves. Saponins, e.g.: acyl virgaurea saponins; clerodane diterpenes, e.g. solidagolactones; phenolic acids	Antiinflammatory, usually in combination, e.g. Phytodolor™. Clinical trial evidence supportive for combined products	0.5–2 g dried herb, as a tea. See manufacturer's instructions for commercial combination products	None known

Goldenseal *Hydrastis canadensis* Extract of root. Isoquinoline alkaloids, e.g. hydrastine, berberine	Antibacterial, antiprotozoal, antidiarrhoeal, digestive. Liver protectant. Some clinical evidence and long history of use	0.7–2 g day dried root/rhizome; 2–4 ml 1:3 tincture, 3.5–7 ml 1:5 tincture. Higher doses used by herbal medicine practitioners for acute conditions	None reported. Extracts of goldenseal inhibit CYP3A4 and displace protein binding to bilirubin in vitro. Berberine and hydrastine inhibit CYP2D6 and CYP3A4 in vitro
Gotu kola (centella, hydrocotyle, Indian pennywort) *Centella asiatica* Extract of herb, taken internally and often applied topically. Saponins, e.g. asiaticoside, madecassoside, brahmoside, centelloside	Use to aid wound healing, burns and other dermatological conditions, and reduce scarring. An important Ayurvedic herb used as an immune stimulant. Some supporting clinical trial evidence, especially for wounds and burns	Internal use: dried herb 0.5–1 g daily or equivalent extract. Topical use: ointment containing, e.g. 10% extract	None reported
Grapeseed *Vitis vinifera* Extract of seed. Proanthocyanidins, catechins, resveratrol	Antioxidant; allergic rhinitis, venous insufficiency. Clinical evidence sparse, but supported by trials on products containing similar constituents (e.g. Pycnogenol™, bilberry, q.v.)	200–500 mg proanthocyanidin-rich extract daily	None reported. Caution with anticancer drugs if taken frequently in high doses

Supplement Compound or herb Botanical or dietary source Type of constituents	Clinical use Traditional and modern, evidence, toxicity, side effects and contraindications	Usual dosage ranges Herb, extract equivalent or doses used in clinical trials	Drug interactions Reports and recommendations based on clinical or sound theoretical grounds
Green tea *Camellia sinensis* Infusion of leaf = tea! Extract of leaf. Caffeine; polyphenols (e.g. epigallocatechin in green tea; theaflavins and thearubigens in black tea); flavonoids	Antioxidant, antimicrobial, chemoprotectant, common refreshing beverage. Green tea is unfermented, black tea is fermented, and Oolong tea is partially fermented. All have antioxidant effects but more evidence for green tea to date	Unrestricted as 'tea', limit of tolerance due to caffeine content. Extract: 1.5–3 g standardized to 50% catechins. Capsules of 100 mg: 1–6 daily	None reported. Catechins inhibit some CYP enzymes and P-gp, but inhibition of CYP enzymes thought to be reason for chemoprotectant effect of tea. Caution with warfarin. Caffeine induces CYP1A2
Guarana *Paullinia cupana* Roasted pulverized seeds. Caffeine (=guaranine), theophylline, theobromine; proanthocyanidins, e.g. catechins	Found in sports supplements and 'tonics'. Stimulant effects due to caffeine	Powdered seeds 0.5–4 g	Caffeine induces CYP1A2. Avoid with other stimulants
Hawthorn *Crataegus oxyacanthoides* [= C. oxyacantha]; C. monogyna. Extracts of leaves with flowers; berries.	Cardiotonic, antioxidant. Increasingly popular herb in Europe and US, for mild heart failure, hypertension and angina	Dried leaf, flower of berry: 1.5–3 g per day. Tablets (made from extract, standardized to 15–20 mg proanthocyanidins	None known. No effect on P-gp but flavonoids can affect some CYP enzymes. Old unconfirmed reports suggest possible

Proanthocyanidins, e.g. catechins; epicatechin dimers; flavonoids, e.g. vitexin, orientin; caffeic acid derivatives	pectoris, improves blood flow; some supporting clinical trial evidence	and 6–7 mg flavonoids); 2–3 times a day; others as directed by product manufacturer. Herbalists use higher doses to control hypertension	potentiation of cardiac glycosides, barbiturates, theophylline and caffeine in animals. Caution with cardiac and antihypertensive drugs
Hops *Humulus lupulus* Flowers (= strobiles). Oleo-resin: α-bitter acids, e.g. humulone, cohumulone; β-bitter acids, e.g. lupulone, adlupulone; essential oil, e.g. humulene; chalcones, e.g. 6-prenylnaringenin	Sedative, often found in combination with other herbs, e.g. passiflora, wild lettuce (q.v.). 6-prenylnaringenin is oestrogenic but not thought to be a problem with normal doses. Use in beer suggests good safety profile!	Dried powdered flowers 0.5 g, or equivalent extract	None known
Horse-chestnut seed *Aesculus hippocastanum* Seed extract. Triterpene saponins, a complex mixture known as aescin (escin)	Main use is for chronic venous insufficiency, especially in lower limbs, oedema and haemorrhoids, with some supporting clinical trial evidence. Antiinflammatory	Dried powdered seed 1–2 g daily. Tablets, e.g. 200 mg extract standardized to 40 mg aescin, 2–3 daily; aescin preparations 100 mg daily. Ointment containing extract	None known

Supplement Compound or herb Botanical or dietary source Type of constituents	Clinical use Traditional and modern, evidence, toxicity, side effects and contraindications	Usual dosage ranges Herb, extract equivalent or doses used in clinical trials	Drug interactions Reports and recommendations based on clinical or sound theoretical grounds
Insect flowers (pyrethrum) *Chrysanthemum cinerariaefolium* and other spp. Flowers. Pyrethroids: pyrethrins, cinerins and jasmolins; sesquiterpene lactones	Insecticide. Used externally to treat head lice and scabies	See manufacturer's instructions	None known
Kava-kava (kava) *Piper methysticum* Extract of root. Pyrones (kava lactones): kawain, methysticin	Withdrawn from market due to rare and idiosyncratic liver toxicity reports. Formerly used for anxiety. Traditionally used as a ceremonial drink in the South Pacific islands	Not recommended	Potent inhibitor of CYP3A4, CYP1A2, CYP2C9, CYP2D6, CYP2C19. Avoid with anticancer drugs and other sedatives
Lapacho (taheebo, pau d'arco) *Tabebuia avellanedae* and others Extract of inner bark. Naphthoquinones, e.g. lapachol, deoxylapachol, lapachones, etc.	Antimicrobial, active against protozoa, bacteria, fungi. Plenty of in vitro evidence but few clinical studies. Traditional use for cancers, but no conclusive clinical evidence for this use, so cannot be recommended	Extract equivalent to 250 mg lapachol, three times daily (as an example only)	None known

Larkspur (consolida) *Delphinium consolida* Extract of seeds. Diterpene alkaloids, e.g. lycoctonine, delconine, delsonine	Antiparasitic. Tincture used externally to treat head lice. These alkaloids are similar to those found in aconite and are very toxic, use with extreme care	Follow manufacturer's instructions	None known
Lemon balm (balm) *Melissa officinalis* Extract of herb. Volatile oil, e.g. citral, caryophyllene, linalool; caffeic acid derivatives	Mild sedative; some clinical evidence and long history of use. Applied topically as an antiviral agent in herpes infections	Dried herb 2–4 g daily or equivalent extract. Tablets containing extract equivalent to approximately 500 mg leaf: three times daily. Topical application: extract up to 10% in ointment base	None known
Lettuce, wild (lettuce opium) *Lactuca virosa* Leaves, dried juice. Sesquiterpene lactones, e.g. lactucin, lactucopicrin, lactuside A; coumarins, e.g. cichoriin, esculentin; flavonoids	Mild sedative and hypnotic, often in combination with hops, passiflora (q.v.). Wide usage but little clinical evidence in support	Dried leaf: 0.5–3 g or equivalent extract, up to three times daily. For combined preparations, see manufacturer's literature	None known. Not thought to be potent enough to interfere with other hypnotic sedatives
Liquorice (licorice) *Glycyrrhiza glabra, G. uralensis* and others. Extract of rhizome ('root').	Antiulcer, antiinflammatory, expectorant, carminative. Wide usage and much supporting evidence, but side	Dried root: 1–4 g; Liquorice Liquid Extract BP 2–5 ml, both up to three times daily	None reported, but may decrease metabolism of other steroids. Extracts affect blood glucose levels and may

102

Supplement Compound or herb Botanical or dietary source Type of constituents	Clinical use Traditional and modern, evidence, toxicity, side effects and contraindications	Usual dosage ranges Herb, extract equivalent or doses used in clinical trials	Drug interactions Reports and recommendations based on clinical or sound theoretical grounds
Triterpenes, e.g. glycyrrhizin (= glycyrrhizic or glycyrrhizinic acid), its aglycone glycyrrhetinic acid (= glycyrrhitic acid) and others; flavonoids, e.g. glabridin, liquiritin and many others; coumarins and polysaccharides	effects show mineralocorticoid activity and include hypertension, hypokalaemia and even Cushing's syndrome. These have been observed more frequently in patients consuming excessive amounts of liquorice confectionary	Dried root: 1–4 g; Liquorice Liquid Extract BP 2–5 ml, both up to three times daily	interfere with hypoglycaemic therapy. Increases activity of some CYP enzymes in rodents after repeated dosing BUT extract shows weak inhibition of CYP3A5 in vitro. Inhibits 5-alpha and 5-beta-reductases, and 11-beta dehydrogenase. Avoid regular, high doses with steroid drugs, including oral contraceptives
Lycopene Carotenoid found in red fruits and vegetables, especially tomato	Antioxidant, chemoprotectant. Epidemiological studies confirm lower cancer risk for high lycopene diet and also reduced cardiovascular disease, but few clinical studies carried out. Not a precursor of vitamin A so very low toxicity	Usually 15–75 mg daily	None known

Ma Huang *Ephedra sinica*, other *Ephedra* spp. Extract of herb. Biogenic amines, e.g. ephedrine, norephedrine, pseudoephedrine; diterpenes, e.g. ephedrannins	Slimming aid, antiasthmatic, decongestant. Liable to abuse; banned from sale in USA. Ephedrine is a sympathomimetic with amfetamine-like effects in large doses	Powdered herb: 1–4 g daily; or equivalent extract; pure ephedrine: 15–60 mg three times daily; ephedrine nose drops 0.5–1%	Potential, theoretical interaction with MAOIs a serious possibility. Avoid use with MAOIs, other stimulants, halothane anaesthetics, anti-arrhythmics and all drugs contraindicated with ephedrine
Marshmallow *Althaea officinalis* Extract of root and herb. Mucilage: composed of polysaccharides of, e.g. L-rhamnose, D-galactose, D-galacturonic acid, etc; flavonoids, etc	Demulcent, antitussive, soothing to irritated mucous membranes. No clinical trial evidence but long history of use. Used to make marshmallow confectionary	Water extract of 2–5 g dried leaf or root, three times daily; poultice applied externally	None known
Meadowsweet (queen of the meadow) *Filipendula ulmaria (Spiraea filipendula)* Extract of flowers, herb. Essential oil, e.g. salicylaldehyde (up to 75%), methyl salicylate; phenolic glycosides, e.g. monotropein, spiraein (hydrolyse to salicylic acid); flavonoids	Antiinflammatory, analgesic. Contains salicylates but ADR profile appears safer than for other salicylate drugs	Dried herb or flowers: 4–6 g daily or equivalent extract	None reported, but avoid with NSAIDs, warfarin, methotrexate, phenytoin, valproate, spironolactone as a precaution

104

Supplement Compound or herb Botanical or dietary source Type of constituents	Clinical use Traditional and modern, evidence, toxicity, side effects and contraindications	Usual dosage ranges Herb, extract equivalent or doses used in clinical trials	Drug interactions Reports and recommendations based on clinical or sound theoretical grounds
Melatonin N-acetyl-5-methoxytryptamine; primary hormone secreted by the pineal gland. Low levels found in bananas and cereals	Used to control circadian rhythm, mainly for sleep disorders and jet-lag; also for 'anti-ageing' and antioxidant properties	0.5–5 mg daily dose, taken at night to induce sleep	Avoid with tranquillizers, antidepressants (especially MAOIs) and warfarin. Not suitable for children (who have naturally high levels), pregnant women or those wishing to conceive, in allergy or autoimmune disease
Milk thistle (St Mary's thistle) *Silybum marianum* Extract of seed, herb. Lignans, the mixture known as 'silymarin' containing, e.g. silybin, silydianin, silychristin	Liver protectant, used to treat hepatitis, alcoholic cirrhosis, etc. Used to detoxify generally and counteract poisoning, especially by toxic fungi (*Amanita phalloides*, etc.). Liver protection has clinical evidence in support	Tablets made of 200 mg extract, standardized to silymarin content of 140 mg: 1–2 daily. 1:1 extract: 5–10 ml. Higher does used in severe liver damage or poisoning	None known. Weak inhibition of P-gp-mediated cellular efflux; little effect on CYP enzymes including CYP3A4, so probably safe with anticancer drugs metabolized by CYP3A4. No interference with pharmacokinetics of indinavir in healthy human subjects

Nettle (stinging nettle) *Urtica dioica* Extract of root or leaf (different indications). Root: lignans, e.g. pinoresinol, secoisolariciresinol; lectins, the mixture known as UDA (Urtica Dioica Agglutinin), composed of at least 6 isolectins; triterpenes, e.g. oleanolic and ursolic acid derivatives. Leaf: flavonoids, quercetin, kaempferol; indoles, e.g. choline, histamine; vitamin K	Root extracts used to treat benign prostate hyperplasia (BPH); there is pharmacological and some clinical evidence in support. Avoid in prostate cancer to avoid masking of symptoms. Often used in combination with saw palmetto and/or pygeum bark (q.v.). Young fresh leaves used as a food, dried leaf extracts used as an antiinflammatory in arthritis. Considered safe (although fresh leaves sting!)	Dr ed root: 4–6 g daily. Clinical trial doses: For BPH, equivalent 5:1 extracts used at doses of 600–1200 mg. Dried leaf or herb: 8–12 g daily. Clinical trial doses: For arthritis, extracts equivalent to about 9 g herb daily	None known
Oats *Avena sativa* Proteins, prolamines known as avenin, avenalin and gliadin; starch and soluble polysaccharides: mainly beta-glucans and arabinogalactans; saponin glycosides, including	Internally used as an antidepressant and cardiac tonic, and for debility and menopausal symptoms. Food use widespread: beneficial effects include lowering blood cholesterol levels.	Dose not confirmed but commercial products use tinctures given as drops. For external use, oats added to the bath	None known nor expected. Oats is a common food

Supplement Compound or herb Botanical or dietary source Type of constituents	Clinical use Traditional and modern, evidence, toxicity, side effects and contraindications	Usual dosage ranges Herb, extract equivalent or doses used in clinical trials	Drug interactions Reports and recommendations based on clinical or sound theoretical grounds
avenacosides A and B, and soyasaponin I; phytosterols: cholesterol, beta-sitosterol, delta-5-avenasterol. Fatty oil, composed of avenoleic, oleic, ricinoleic and linoleic acids; vitamin E, vitamin B	External use as an emollient in dry skin diseases such as eczema and psoriasis		
Octosanol and policosanol A 28-carbon aliphatic alcohol found in whole grains, and surface waxy layer of many fruits and leaves. Policosanol is a mixture of primary alcohols extracted from sugar cane, the main constituent of which is octosanol	Enhancement of athletic performance; Parkinson's and motor neurone diseases; hypercholesterolaemia; improvement of platelet function. Some clinical evidence but not conclusive yet. Good safety profile and well tolerated	Variable, usually 5–10 mg, occasionally up to 40 mg, daily	None known

Oregon grape (mountain grape) *Berberis aquifolium (Mahonia aquifolium)* Extract of root and rhizome. Benzylisoquinoline alkaloids, e.g. berberine, oxyberberine, berbamine, oxyacanthine; aporphine alkaloids, e.g. isocoydine, isothebaine, magnoflorine	Antiseptic, digestive, liver protectant. Used for diarrhoea, gastric disorders, and especially for skin diseases such as psoriasis and acne, where it may be applied topically. Pharmacological and some clinical evidence in support	Dried root: 1–2 g or equivalent extract	None known. Berberine and hydrastine inhibit CYP2D6 and CYP3A4 in vitro
Ornithine alpha ketoglutarate A dietary amino acid precursor of glutamine, arginine, polyamines, etc.	Enhances tissue repair, protein synthesis. Used to aid healing in burn injury and after surgery and for wasting diseases, with supporting evidence. Taken by athletes but no evidence of improved performance yet. Safety profile good	10–30 g daily, in divided doses	No interactions known. Some diarrhoea reported with very high doses

108

Supplement Compound or herb Botanical or dietary source Type of constituents	Clinical use Traditional and modern, evidence, toxicity, side effects and contraindications	Usual dosage ranges Herb, extract equivalent or doses used in clinical trials	Drug interactions Reports and recommendations based on clinical or sound theoretical grounds
Passiflora (passionflower) *Passiflora incarnate, P. edulis* Herb extract. Flavonoids, e.g. chrysin, orientin, isovitexin, schaftoside, isochaftoside, saponaretin; alkaloids, e.g. tetrahydrocarbolines (presence of harman, harmaline, harmine, etc. disputed)	Mild sedative and hypnotic. Some pharmacological evidence now emerging to support usage, but little clinical evidence to date. Generally considered safe. *P. edulis* fruits are edible (= passion fruit)	Dried herb 0.25–1 g, or equivalent extract	None known
Pelargonium (Umckaloabo™) *Pelargonium sidoides* Herb extract. Polyphenols, e.g. catechin, gallocatechin, and gallic acid) and coumarins (e.g., umckalin); simple phenolics	Antiviral for use in colds and influenza, bronchitis, coughs, upper respiratory tract irritation, and gastrointestinal complaints. Clinical evidence mounting to support use. A product made from the root ('Steven's Cure') was popular in England as a cure for tuberculosis in the late 19th century	Tablets containing 2 mg dry extract, three or four times daily for up to 10 days; liquid extract 1.5 ml three times daily, children 6–12 years 1 ml dose (for tonsillitis, etc.)	None known but avoid with warfarin as a precaution

Peppermint *Mentha x piperita* Oil; leaf extract. Oil: menthol, menthone, menthyl acetate, menthofuran, piperitone, and others. Herb: oil as above, and flavonoids, e.g. menthoside, rutin; caffeic acid derivatives	Carminative, digestive, decongestant, coolant. Oil, in enteric-coated capsules, used for IBS. Menthol used as an inhalation for congested airways in colds, etc. Very wide usage including in foods and confectionary; considered safe, but pure oil must be used with caution and in small amounts	Powdered herb 2–4 g or equivalent extract, up to three times a day. Oil: 0.05–2 ml. Concentrated Peppermint Water BPC 1973: 0.25–1 ml	None known. Inhibition of P-gp by extract and possibly oil
Pumpkin seed *Cucurbita pepo* Seeds of soft shell varieties; isolated sterol mixture. Phytosterols, e.g. spirostanol, cholestane and lathostanol derivatives; linoleic, oleic acids	Benign prostate hyperplasia (BPH). Some clinical evidence to support usage, long-term use required for effects, no adverse effects noted. Often used in combination with saw palmetto, nettle root, pygeum bark (q.v.)	90 mg daily of isolated sterol mixture	None known

Supplement Compound or herb Botanical or dietary source Type of constituents	Clinical use Traditional and modern, evidence, toxicity, side effects and contraindications	Usual dosage ranges Herb, extract equivalent or doses used in clinical trials	Drug interactions Reports and recommendations based on clinical or sound theoretical grounds
Pycnogenol™ (pine bark extract) *Pinus maritima* Extract of bark. Polyphenols, e.g. catechin, epicatechin; proanthocyanidins and procyanidins	Antioxidant and antithrombotic; used for traveller's thrombosis and various inflammatory, ageing and degenerative disorders. Antidiabetic and free radical scavenger. Applied topically to aid wound healing and prevent scarring. Some clinical evidence available for most indications	50–300 mg extract daily, depending on indication; gel containing 1% applied topically	None known
Pygeum bark *Prunus africana (Pygeum africanum)* Lipophilic extract of bark. Sterols and pentacyclic triterpenes, e.g. oleanolic, ursolic, abietic and crataegolic acids	Benign prostate hyperplasia (BPH). Pharmacological and some clinical evidence to support usage, long-term use required for effects, no adverse effects noted. Often used in combination with saw palmetto (q.v.)	100–200 mg lipophilic extract daily	None known

Raspberry leaf
Rubus idaeus
Infusion of leaves.
Flavonoids, e.g. rutin, kaempferol, but actives largely unknown

Facilitation of childbirth. An infusion is drunk throughout pregnancy. Clinical evidence from 2 studies is conflicting, there are no toxicity data but the clinical studies showed no adverse effects

Dried leaf 4–8 g three times daily

Red clover
Trifolium pratense
Extract of dried flowers, herb.
Isoflavones, e.g. genistein, biochanin A, daidzein, afrormosin, formononetin, pratensin and others; coumarins, e.g. coumestrol, medicagol; clovamides

Phyto-oestrogen, now used as a natural HRT; traditionally used for skin complaints. Little clinical evidence for skin disorders (but long history of use), more evidence available for HRT claims, supported by other trials of isoflavones (e.g. soya, q.v.), which also increase bone density. Considered safe, but use of phyto-oestrogens in women with history of breast cancer not recommended until more data available

Dried herb or flowers 4 g three times daily, or equivalent extract.
Isoflavone extract: 50–150 mg daily or more

No clinical reports. Red clover extract inhibits CYP3A4, and genistein inhibits several CYP enzymes in vitro and interacts with P-gp and other transporters. Theoretical considerations suggest avoidance with HRT, also tamoxifen and other treatments for breast cancer

Supplement Compound or herb Botanical or dietary source Type of constituents	Clinical use Traditional and modern, evidence, toxicity, side effects and contraindications	Usual dosage ranges Herb, extract equivalent or doses used in clinical trials	Drug interactions Reports and recommendations based on clinical or sound theoretical grounds
Red vine leaf *Vitis vinifera* Extract of leaf. Flavonoids including quercetin-3-O-beta-D-glucuronide and isoquercitrin	Chronic venous insufficiency, oedema, 'heavy legs'	360–720 mg daily of commercial standardized extract AS 195 used in clinical studies	None known
Red yeast rice, fermented rice 'cholestin' *Monascus purpureus* Fermentation product of rice. A series of monocolins, including monacolin K (mevinolin or lovastatin), J, L, M, X, and their hydroxy acid form, as well as dehydromonacolin K, dihydromonacolin L, compactin, 3-alpha-hydroxy-3,5-dihydromonacolin L, etc.	Natural source of statins, e.g. lovastatin. Reduces hepatic cholesterol synthesis, used in the same way as pharmaceutical statins such as simvastatin	Proprietary product 'cholestin' usually taken at 1.2 g twice daily but variation in natural product complicates dosage titration	May cause similar adverse reactions as other statins, e.g. rhabdomyolysis; anaphylaxis has been reported

113

Rhodiola *Rhodiola rosea* Root extract. Phenylpropanoids, e.g. rosavin, rosin, rosarin; phenylethanol derivatives, e.g. salidroside (rhodioloside), tyrosol; flavonoids, e.g. rodiolin, rodionin; monoterpenes, e.g. rosiridol, rosaridin sterols; caffeic acid derivatives	Increasingly popular adaptogen and stimulant, used for stress and fatigue. Clinical evidence available in support of usage; safety tests show lack of toxicity. Recent use also for erectile dysfunction, cardioprotection; more research needed	Extract of root, standardized for phenylpropanoids (3%, calculated as rosavin) and phenylethanols (1%, as salidroside), e.g. Rosavin™: dose 100–300 mg daily	None known, but may have additive effects with other stimulants
Rhubarb *Rheum emodi, R. palmatum*, etc. Root and rhizome. Anthraquinones, e.g. chrysophanic acid, emodin, aloe-emodin, rhein and their glucosides; tannins and procyanidins; stilbenes, e.g. rhaponticin, resveratrol	Well-known stimulant anthraquinone laxative, but paradoxically used in Chinese medicine as a digestive and astringent. Should not be taken for long periods. Avoid in obstructive bowel disorders	Dried root and rhizome: 0.2–1 g three times daily or equivalent extract	None reported. Avoid regular use with thiazide diuretics and corticosteroids to prevent electrolyte imbalance
Rosemary *Rosmarinus officinalis* Herb extract, essential oil. Caffeic acid derivatives, e.g. rosmarinic, chlorogenic, neochlorogenic and caffeic acids; flavonoids, e.g. apigenin, diosmin, genkwanin; volatile oil, e.g. borneol, camphor, cineole, linalool	Increasingly popular as a memory enhancer, with some pharmacological and clinical evidence in support. Oil is stimulant and antiseptic, used in aromatherapy; should not be taken internally and avoided in pregnant women	Dried herb 2–4 g daily or equivalent extract	None known. In vitro inhibition of P-gp

Supplement Compound or herb Botanical or dietary source Type of constituents	Clinical use Traditional and modern, evidence, toxicity, side effects and contraindications	Usual dosage ranges Herb, extract equivalent or doses used in clinical trials	Drug interactions Reports and recommendations based on clinical or sound theoretical grounds
St John's wort *Hypericum perforatum* Total herb extract. Naphthodianthrones known as hypericins, e.g. hypericin, pseudohypericin, protohypericin, protopseudohypericin, cyclo pseudohypericin; hyperforin and adhyperforin; flavonoids, e.g. hyperin, rutin; volatile oil (<1%)	Mild to moderate depression; seasonal affective disorder. Important and popular herb with much anecdotal and clinical evidence, some of which is disputed. Products highly variable in composition and quality. For external use, macerated flowers in olive oil used traditionally to aid wound healing. Good safety profile despite interaction potential	Extract (standardized for hypericin and hyperforin content) 200–1800 mg daily. Usual dose in clinical trials has been 900 mg daily and is considered equivalent to most synthetic antidepressants. 2–3 g dried herb, as herbal tea	High potential for interaction. Significant induction of CYPs 2E1, 3A4, 1A2, 2D6, 2C19. Competing effects on P-gp: initially inhibited then induced. Conflicting reports on theophylline: interaction reported, but SJW did not affect serum levels of theophylline (via CYP1A2) in human volunteers. Avoid with anticoagulants, oral contraceptives, immune suppressants, digoxin, opiates, antineoplastics, protease inhibitors, fexofenadine, statins, omeprazole, verapamil and other antidepressants

Sage
Salvia officinalis, S. lavandulifolia
Extract of herb; oil.
Caffeic acid derivatives, e.g. salvianolic, rosmarinic, labiatic and caffeic acids; flavonoids, e.g. salvigenin, luteolin, genkwanin; volatile oil, e.g. thujone, borneol camphor, cineole, linalool; diterpenes, e.g. royleanones, picrosalvin; salviatannin

Increasingly popular as a memory enhancer; some pharmacological and clinical evidence. Mouthwash or gargle in throat infections. Oil is stimulant and antiseptic. *Salvia lavandulifolia* preferred to *S. officinalis* (the former does not contain toxic thujone)

Dried herb 1–4 g daily or equivalent extract. Tablets containing high-quality leaf: 300 mg three times daily

None known

Saw palmetto (sabal)
Serenoa repens (= *Sabal serrulata*)
Lipophilic extract of seed.
Fixed oil with approximately 25% fatty acids, e.g. lauric, palmitic, capric, caprylic, oleic, linoleic and linolenic acids; sterols, e.g. beta-sitosterol; long chain alcohols, e.g. farnesol, phytol

Used in benign prostate hyperplasia, with good clinical evidence. Constituents are commonplace and safe but avoid in suspected prostate cancer to prevent masking of symptoms
Often used in combination with nettle and/or pygeum bark (q.v.)

Powdered berries 0.5–1 g daily or ecuivalent extract; commercial lipophilic extract 320 mg daily

None known. Absence of effect on CYP3A4 and CYP2D6. (Some authorities recommend avoidance with hormonal therapies but without clinical evidence.)

115

116

Supplement Compound or herb Botanical or dietary source Type of constituents	Clinical use Traditional and modern, evidence, toxicity, side effects and contraindications	Usual dosage ranges Herb, extract equivalent or doses used in clinical trials	Drug interactions Reports and recommendations based on clinical or sound theoretical grounds
Schisandra *Schisandra chinensis* Extract of fruit (berry). Lignans, several series including, e.g. schisandrins, schizandrols, schisantherins, (also known as gomisins and wuweizisus)	Chinese herb becoming more popular world-wide. An 'adaptogen' used to improve physical and mental stamina; some supporting clinical trial evidence. Liver protectant	1.5–6 g powdered fruits daily or equivalent extract	None known. Potentiates effects of neuroleptics, barbiturates and benzodiazepines in some animal models. Caution with other CNS drugs
Senna *Cassia angustifolia, C. senna* Fruit (pods) and leaf; extracts and infusions. Anthraquinones, e.g. sennosides A, B, C, D, etc; aloe-emodin, palmidin A, rhein anthrone and their glucosides and others	Widely used stimulant anthraquinone laxative. Should not be taken for long periods, may cause dependence. Avoid in obstructive bowel disorders. May be used combined with a bulk laxative, e.g. ispaghula, in products such as Manevac™. Formerly used during pregnancy but no longer recommended	Senna tablets BP, containing 7.5 mg standardized extract (calculated as sennoside B), dose 1–2 at night. Powdered leaf or fruit: 0.5–2 g as a tea, for occasional use only	None reported. Excessive intake can cause hypokalaemia and enhance toxicity of cardiac glycosides. AQs interact with CYP enzymes as substrates, inducers and inhibitors but overall effect unpredictable. Avoid regular use with thiazide diuretics and corticosteroids to prevent electrolyte imbalance

117

Soya *Glycine max* Isoflavone extract of beans; powdered beans used as food. Isoflavones, e.g. genistein, daidzein, glycetin; protein. Soya food (tofu, soya milk, tempeh, etc.) contains isoflavones, but processed soya protein has very little	Phyto-oestrogen used as a natural HRT; clinical evidence increasing and supported by other trials of isoflavones (e.g. red clover, q.v.), which also increase bone density. Considered safe, but use of phyto-oestrogens in women with history of breast cancer not recommended until more data available. Soya protein (25 g daily) lowers blood cholesterol; soya 'milk' used as a substitute for daily in lactose/milk intolerance	Isoflavone extract: 50–150 mg daily or more. One glass soya milk supposedly equivalent to 50 mg isoflavones. Average dietary intake in the US is 1–2 mg (calculated as genistein); 20–80 mg in Japan. Soya protein: 10 g contains approx 50 mg isoflavones; dietary supplement usually about 10–25 g daily	No clinical reports, and conflicting evidence between effects of genistein, an isolated ingredient, and the total extract of soya. Genistein inhibits various CYP enzymes and P-gp, but soya extract does NOT affect CYP3A4. Theoretical considerations suggest avoidance with HRT, also tamoxifen and other treatments for breast cancer
Spirulina/blue green algae *Spirulina platensis, S. maxima* and others. Cyanobacteria isolated from alkaline lakes. Protein 60–70%, lipids 9–14%, mainly gammalinolenic acid, beta-carotene, minerals	Marketed as a food supplement to lower cholesterol, improve immune function, reduce risks of cancer, etc. None proven but constituents probably do have some benefits	3–10 g algae daily. Capsules available containing, e.g., 500 mg	None known

118

Supplement Compound or herb Botanical or dietary source Type of constituents	Clinical use Traditional and modern, evidence, toxicity, side effects and contraindications	Usual dosage ranges Herb, extract equivalent or doses used in clinical trials	Drug interactions Reports and recommendations based on clinical or sound theoretical grounds
Starflower (borage) oil *Borago officinalis* Seed oil. Gammalinolenic acid (GLA), linoleic and other acids	Used in a similar way to evening primrose oil (q.v.)	2–4 g daily	See evening primrose oil. The leaves of the plants contain toxic pyrrolizidine alkaloids, but these do not occur in the seed oil
Tea tree oil *Melaleuca alternifolia* Essential oil distilled from fresh leaves and twigs. Terpinen-4-ol, cineole, terpineol, etc.	Antiseptic, antiinflammatory, insecticide. Applied topically to the skin for insect bites, wounds, lice, scabies and infections, and to the hair for head lice and dandruff	Can be applied externally undiluted (unlike most essential oils) to lesions only; use sparingly. Good-quality oil (i.e. high terpinene-4-ol containing) not usually irritant	None known
Thyme *Thymus vulgaris* Essential oil distilled from herb; extract of herb	Respiratory disorders, as an expectorant and broncholytic. Thymol is a powerful antiseptic and used in dentistry as an ingredient of toothpastes and mouthwashes	Herb (as an infusion) 1–4 g or equivalent extract. Essential oil and thymol not suitable for internal use except in very small doses as part of a combined preparation (e.g. throat lozenge, cough mixture)	None known

119

Tolu balsam *Myroxylon balsamum* Resin extruded from incisions in the bark. Cinnamic and benzoic acids, benzyl benzoate, their esters with coniferyl alcohol, etc.	Expectorant, stimulant, antiseptic. Used in cough mixtures and steam inhalations for respiratory disorders; applied in creams and ointments as skin protector and antiseptic, especially for prevention of pressure sores. An ingredient of Friar's Balsam	Can be applied externally undiluted but usually 10% in a topical base. Internal use tincture 1:10; 2–4 ml	None known. Can cause allergic reactions in susceptible individuals
Turmeric *Curcuma longa* Powdered rhizome ('root') and extract. Diarylheptanoids, curcuminoids, e.g. curcumin, desmethoxycurcumin, bisdesmethoxycurcumin; essential oil, e.g. turmerone, zingiberene, sabinene	Used to treat rheumatism, infections, and liver disorders (avoid in cases of gallstones). Antiinflammatory and antioxidant. Reduces cholesterol, cancer chemopreventant. Important Ayurvedic and Chinese herb, and popular spice and colourant used in cooking	4–8 g dried rhizome daily, can be mixed with water to form a slurry. Lecithin improves absorption. Liquid extract 1:1 5–15 ml daily in divided doses	None known. Curcumin inhibits P-gp, but has very poor oral bio-availability. Caution in patients taking high doses with anticoagulants or antiplatelet drugs

Supplement Compound or herb Botanical or dietary source Type of constituents	Clinical use Traditional and modern, evidence, toxicity, side effects and contraindications	Usual dosage ranges Herb, extract equivalent or doses used in clinical trials	Drug interactions Reports and recommendations based on clinical or sound theoretical grounds
Valerian *Valerian officinalis* Extract of root. Iridoids: valpotriates, e.g. valtrate, isovaltrate, didrovaltrate; sesquiterpenes, e.g. valerenic acid, valerenone; GABA; essential oil. NB. Valepotriates labile, decompose to valeric acid derivatives	Insomnia, stress, anxiety. Widely used, with clinical evidence to support effects (but not as potent as synthetic hypnotic sedatives) and few 'hangover' effects reported. No serious overdoses or toxicity reported despite years of use. Valerian has an unpleasant smell and is usually taken in tablet form	Dried root: 0.3–1g up to three times daily. Extract: for insomnia, 200–1000 mg (usually 400 mg) about an hour before bedtime. Lower doses used during the day for stress or anxiety	No clinical reports involving sedative interactions. Extract weakly inhibits CYP3A4, CYP2D6 and CYP2C19 and may potentiate effects of barbiturates and chlorpromazine in animals. Multiple night-time doses had minimal effect on CYP3A4 and no effect on CYP2D6 activity in human volunteers
Vervain (verbena) *Verbena officinalis* Infusion of herb (tea) or extract. Iridoids, e.g. verbenalin, aucubin, verbascoside; essential oil, e.g. verbenone, citral; triterpenes; flavonoids	Sedative, tonic, coughs and colds. Little clinical trial evidence but long history of use	Dried herb 2–4 g three times daily or equivalent extract	None known

White horehound
Marrubium vulgare
Extract of herb.
Labdane diterpenes, e.g. marrubiin, premarrubiin, marrubiol, sclareol; alkaloids, e.g. betonicine; volatile oil

Expectorant, antiasthmatic. Used in cough mixtures and particularly in bronchitis. Little clinical trial evidence but long history of use

Dried herb 1–2 g three times daily or equivalent extract

None known

Wild yam
Dioscorea villosa
Steroidal saponins based on diosgenin, e.g. dioscin, dioscorin

Antiinflammatory, used traditionally for intestinal colic. Recent usage as a form of hormone replacement therapy (steroidal saponins are biogenic precursors of sex hormones) as tablets and a cream. However, no evidence for this use or that percutaneous absorption occurs. Mainly used as source of steroids for the pharmaceutical industry

As an antiinflammatory (traditional use) dried root or rhizome 2–4 g as a decoction, three times daily or equivalent extract

None known. May theoretically increase blood levels of endogenous steroid hormones

Supplement Compound or herb Botanical or dietary source Type of constituents	Clinical use Traditional and modern, evidence, toxicity, side effects and contraindications	Usual dosage ranges Herb, extract equivalent or doses used in clinical trials	Drug interactions Reports and recommendations based on clinical or sound theoretical grounds
Willow bark *Salix alba* and other spp. Extract of bark. Phenolic glycosides, e.g. salicin, picein, esters of salicylic acid and salicyl alcohol and derivatives	Antiinflammatory, analgesic. Originally used to provide a source of aspirin. Clinical evidence to support effects and ADR profile appears safer than for other salicylates	Dried bark, as a decoction or extract, 2–4 g three times daily	No clinical reports, but avoid with other NSAIDs, warfarin, methotrexate, phenytoin, valproate, spironolactone as a precaution
Wormwood (absinthe) *Artemisia absinthium* Infusion of herb. Essential oil containing thujone, thujyl alcohol, azulenes; sesquiterpene lactones, e.g. absinthin, artemetin, absintholides	Bitter digestive stimulant and tonic, anthelminthic. Stimulates saliva production and bile flow; used to promote appetite. Used to prepare the liqueur 'absinthe' which is toxic in large doses (due to thujone content) but teas not thought to be harmful	1–2 g herb as an infusion (tea)	None known. Oil should not be used internally: thujone causes hallucinations and mental disorders if used over a long period

NB: Entries marked 'none known' do not necessarily imply negative results, but have mainly not been tested.

CHAPTER 3

Homeopathy and aromatherapy

INTRODUCTION

Homeopathy (also spelled homoeopathy) and aromatherapy have been grouped together in this section because, although their principles and scientific basis (if any) are very different, they could be considered as relevant to pharmacists in a similar fashion. Consumers will often purchase their remedy of choice – a homeopathic remedy or an essential oil – from a pharmacy *without* consulting the pharmacist or asking for advice. Commonly, the general public does not consider intervention by the pharmacist to be important for CAM, and to some extent this may be appropriate. However, as with supplying all forms of over-the-counter (OTC) medication, it may be necessary to identify any suspected serious illness which should be referred to a doctor. Pharmacological interactions between medical prescriptions, OTC drugs and homeopathic remedies or externally applied essential oils may be unlikely but other adverse reactions, such as allergic reactions to essential oils, may occur.

In the case of homeopathy, molecular concentrations of 'drug' in the remedy are very low, or indeed theoretically absent, due to the amount of dilution involved in the homeopathic process. The essential oil components associated with aromatherapy, although known to be absorbed through the skin, tend to only occur in very low amounts and in some instances are the same substances found in culinary herbs and spices (see also herbalism) and so are generally considered safe enough to be sold OTC. The scientific basis for these therapies has yet to be substantiated and claims concerning efficacy continue to be contested. In the case of homeopathy, the premises are in fact incompatible with scientific theory, whereas in aromatherapy it is a question of the actual dose reaching the bloodstream, and an understanding of the effect of olfaction on parts of the brain (psychoneuropharmacology).

Homeopathy

Scientifically, homeopathy is probably the most controversial of all common forms of CAM. However, it is very well established and popular with patients. For that reason alone, it is necessary for pharmacists to familiarize themselves with the basic principles and most common remedies. Despite the lack of scientific evidence, there is a widespread belief in its efficacy and homeopathy is even practised in veterinary medicine, where the placebo effect is unlikely to be acting. It is described as a complete system of healing, offering a philosophy for health and illness, together with a distinct approach to the diagnosis and treatment of a wide range of complaints and disorders. Homeopathy (closely followed by aromatherapy) is now the most widely used alternative system of medicine in the UK, Europe, USA, Canada and Australia (see Box 3.1).

Aromatherapy

Aromatherapy, the topical use of essential (volatile) oils to provide therapeutic effects, is a very popular and common form of alternative medicine. Whilst it is presented as a discrete therapeutic entity, it has also been widely adopted by the beauty and cosmetics industry. This has contributed to the view of aromatherapy as harmless.

However, it is increasingly being shown in clinical studies to have therapeutic benefits. The pharmacological

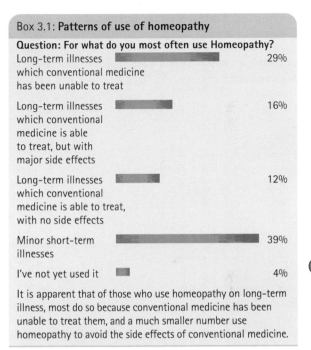

Box 3.1: **Patterns of use of homeopathy**

Question: For what do you most often use Homeopathy?

Long-term illnesses which conventional medicine has been unable to treat	29%
Long-term illnesses which conventional medicine is able to treat, but with major side effects	16%
Long-term illnesses which conventional medicine is able to treat, with no side effects	12%
Minor short-term illnesses	39%
I've not yet used it	4%

It is apparent that of those who use homeopathy on long-term illness, most do so because conventional medicine has been unable to treat them, and a much smaller number use homeopathy to avoid the side effects of conventional medicine.

Adapted from ABC Homoeopathy (www.abchomeopathy.com)

properties of essential oils are well documented and it has been demonstrated that essential oil components are absorbed through the skin and can be measured in the breath around 20 minutes after topical administration. However, it is not necessarily the case that topical application of essential oils gives rise to therapeutic blood levels or that the effect mirrors exactly the effects of ingestion, since different constituents may be differently absorbed.

Although it is often said that aromatherapy originated with the ancient Egyptians, there is no real evidence for this. More likely this is one of the earliest recorded depictions of its use, which is another matter. Certainly the practice of using essential oils, balsams and resins as perfumes or incense, and preservatives in embalming, can hardly be construed as therapeutic. Aromatherapy is actually a fairly recent introduction, as will be discussed later.

Homeopathy

> *Principles:* works on the principle that 'like treats like', i.e. an illness is treated with a medicine which could produce similar symptoms in a healthy person; active ingredients are given in highly diluted form to avoid toxicity
>
> *Positive aspects:* wide-ranging application, including the elderly and infants; no apparent interaction with conventional drugs
>
> *Negative aspects:* scientific rationale unexplained; evidence of efficacy limited and many scientists attribute any successes to placebo effect. Abreactions rare but may occur although no scientific rationale for this

Development and general principles of homeopathy

The discipline was founded in 1796 by Samuel Hahnemann, a German physician and apothecary. At the time, medical practice was often harsh and deaths due to treatment (rather than the disease) were commonplace. The use of highly toxic heavy metals (such as arsenic and mercury), bloodletting (by incisions or leeches) and the administration of strong purgatives and emetics were widespread.

Hahnemann was reputedly disillusioned with these treatments and gave up practising medicine for a while. During this period, he translated medical books and found himself in disagreement with an account of the effects of cinchona bark, which was successfully used to treat malaria. While experimenting on himself by taking high doses of cinchona, he experienced symptoms similar to those of malaria and so began to reduce the dose to try to avoid the unwanted side effects, and is alleged to have found that the efficacy was unchanged but the treatment much safer. Hahnemann then experimented with healthy volunteers who were given many other drugs and other substances in order to build up a 'symptom picture' for each. He referred to this as a 'proving' and this method of evaluating homeopathic remedies continues today. No testing on animals occurs.

On the basis of these findings, Hahnemann outlined three basic principles of homeopathy, still considered valid today, and which form the basis of classical homeopathy.

- 'Like cures like'
- The minimum dose must be used; dilution increases potency
- Only a single remedy or substance should be used in a patient at any one time

Explanation and comments

1. 'Like cures like' or 'Similia similibus curentur'

■ This is a basic tenet of homeopathy (and it also explains the name: *homo* meaning 'like' and *pathos* meaning 'suffering'). Put simply, it means that a substance which, in large doses, causes symptoms in a healthy person can be used, in low doses, to treat those same symptoms in a person who is ill. For example, Rhus tox, derived from poison ivy (botanical name, *Rhus toxicodendron*), which causes a blistering, itchy rash, would be used to treat chicken pox.

Comment: *in an attempt to justify homeopathy, it has been suggested that there are some comparisons with vaccination, in that exposure to a small (or at least survivable) dose of an infective agent will confer immunity (i.e. the opposite effect to causing disease). It has also been said that there are similarities to the process of desensitization, which may be done in patients with allergies to dust mites, grass pollen and other allergens. It is also well known that some conventional drugs, particularly hormones, have the opposite effect when given at a different dose. However, in neither case is a comparison valid since* **measurable** *doses are* *always involved in allopathic medicine. Even if there were any substance in these ideas, they do not fit with the idea of serial dilution and potentization as shown below. More recently, it has been suggested that 'the length of the bond between molecules increases in length with repetitive succession sites' (Kirkman 2004). This has no supporting scientific evidence or rationale.*

2. The use of minimum doses: the concept of potentization

■ Hahnemann developed a method of serial dilution which allowed poisonous substances to be administered safely. He called this 'potentization' and it involved both dilution of the substance and vigorous shaking during this process, which he referred to as 'succussion'. Basically, it means that the more the remedy is diluted, the more potent it becomes. Many homeopathic preparations are so highly diluted that they are statistically unlikely to contain a single molecule of the starting material.

129

Comment: *dilution and succussion are considered by homeopaths to be an important method of harnessing and increasing the properties of a remedy, and it is still how homeopathic medicines are made today (although the shaking is usually done mechanically). It is a fiercely disputed concept since homeopaths claim that the more diluted the remedy, the more potent it becomes, due to the process of succussion. It is difficult for a pharmacist to accept this, as it is the opposite of current scientific thinking. The concept of adding a form of 'energy' during such a process is not usually considered a factor in increasing therapeutic properties, although there are scientific phenomena which can be used in the argument. For example, it is well known that energy may need to be added in the form of heat (or shaking) to dissolve substances, and also that energy in the form of heat is liberated when concentrated acids are diluted with water. Unfortunately, these examples are hardly analogous since after the initial dilution, little energy change is observed. In response to the claim that the remedy contains none of the starting material, and* *therefore cannot have an effect, some homeopaths have compared the idea of conventional analysis of homeopathic medicines, i.e. chemical analysis, to be like describing a computer disk in terms of the amount of plastic or metal in it: it gives no indication of the amount of information contained in such a disk. Another theory postulates that the medium (usually water) retains an 'imprint' of the original molecule. These are analogies, not scientific theories.*

3. **Only a single remedy or substance should be used in a patient at any one time**
■ No matter how many symptoms are experienced, usually only one remedy is taken and that remedy will be aimed at all those symptoms.

Comment: *in recent years, homeopathic remedies have been sold increasingly as combinations designed for self-medication, and it is also becoming more common for homeopaths to prescribe multiple remedies. A group of remedies, effective in tackling a condition in a range of people, may also be combined in a single pill. This is in contrast to the principles of classical homeopathy. Many homeopaths do not approve of these 'off-the-peg' combinations and consider that there is no substitute for comparing the symptom pictures properly or, if necessary, undergoing an in-depth consultation to identify the correct single remedy for that patient.*

Choosing and dispensing homeopathic remedies

In choosing a remedy, a homeopath will consider the patient's physical, mental and emotional symptoms as well as personal appearance, temperament, likes and dislikes (see Box 3.2). This 'symptom picture' is then matched to that of a homeopathic remedy, often nowadays using a computer program (see Table 3.1). In addition to the basic principles mentioned above, homeopaths believe that homeopathic remedies work by stimulating the body's own healing activity rather than by acting directly on the disease process. It is

Box 3.2: **Examples of questions used in finding the appropriate homeopathic remedy**

Homeopathy relies on prescribing remedies to your precise combination of symptoms, so all must be included in the process. Most of us also have a few long-standing, minor irritations that we rarely notice any more (e.g. poor circulation, leading to cold hands or feet). These should also be included, even if they hardly count as symptoms.
Aside from the obvious nature of the complaint, e.g. headache, things to note include the following.

Symptoms
- When did symptoms first occur, and what brought them on?
- What makes a particular symptom feel worse or better?
- Where exactly is each problem located?

Personal characteristics
- State of mind (including fears, anxieties, attitudes, etc.)
- Your sleep pattern
- Sensitivities, e.g. to light, cold, heat, touch, criticism, etc.
- Colour and consistency and regularity of your stool
- For women, where you are on your monthly cycle

thought that the symptoms of disease represent the efforts of the body to restore health and thus by adding a remedy with the same symptom profile, the healing process is enhanced. Illness is thought to be a consequence of the body's inability to cope with external and emotional factors such as poor diet, stress and adverse environmental conditions, and is therefore different for each individual, so treatment must be chosen on an individual basis. Homeopathy is one of the most holistic of medical systems.

Comment: *conventional medicine is sometimes referred to as 'allopathic' medicine, meaning treatment with opposites, i.e. a fever is treated with an antipyretic, designed to reduce the temperature. The different approaches can be compared by considering the treatment of an infectious disease such as influenza, where the body* *will often respond to a bacterial or other infection with a rise in temperature, i.e. a fever. Although a higher temperature may actually help to kill the infecting agent, excessively high temperatures are uncomfortable and may precipitate fits, especially in children, so in conventional medicine a high temperature will be treated with paracetamol or ibuprofen, for example. In homeopathy, however, a fever may be treated with Lachesis, Belladonna, Bryonia or other remedy, depending on the symptoms. The idea of illness being the result of poor diet, stress and adverse environmental conditions is now accepted by both homeopathic and conventional doctors, but the approach to treatment is the opposite.*

The dose and preparation of remedies: dilution, succussion and potentization

132

A liquid extract of the substance (such as crude plant material, snake venom or metal salt), known as a 'mother tincture', is the starting point for the production of most homeopathic remedies. This is then diluted with vigorous shaking (succussing) according to either a decimal scale, in which dilution steps of 1 in 10 (the D or X potencies) are made, or a centesimal scale, where the dilution is in steps of 1 in 100 (C potencies). These potencies are usually prepared robotically. The centesimal scale is most often used and taking it as an example, the first step involves 1 part of mother tincture being added to 99 parts of diluent to produce a 1 in 100 dilution, known as 1C. The second step involves 1 part of the 1C dilution being added to 99 parts of diluent, producing a 1 in 10,000 dilution (2C).

The most commonly used products are 6C and 30C, and these are found in many pharmacies. These are the potencies recommended for self-medication or acute diseases, whereas the higher dilutions, for example 1M (1 in 10^{2000} dilution, i.e. 2000 centesimal dilution steps) and 10M (1 in $10^{20,000}$) are recommended for use only by qualified practitioners and for more serious or chronic disorders. There are also LM potencies which involve serial dilutions of 1 in 50,000 at each step. From these potentized liquids, pills, tablets and other dosage forms can be made.

According to Hahnemann's second principle, the more dilute the preparation, the more potent it is. So, for example, a 30C remedy is believed to be stronger than a 6C remedy. Also, although 2D and 1C preparations are technically the same concentration, a 2D is considered to be more potent because it has undergone two succussion steps, whereas a 1C preparation has undergone only one.

Self-selection or recommendation by the non-expert

Without further specialist training, the pharmacist belongs firmly in this category. The tables and boxes provided will help in the process of selection of an appropriate remedy but be warned that this can be a time-consuming business not to be attempted in the middle of a busy surgery! As with all recommendations, in the event of a serious illness or lack of diagnosis, the pharmacist should direct the patient to his or her GP; in long-standing illness or for a complex pattern of symptoms, the patient should consult a qualified homeopath.

The role of the pharmacist

In exactly the same way as with conventional medicine, pharmacists may be required to give advice for minor ailments, sell over-the-counter remedies or dispense prescriptions written by a medical doctor or registered homeopath. Nowadays a small but increasing percentage of practitioners hold both qualifications.

OTC sales and advice

Most pharmacies carry a range of homeopathic remedies, usually 6C or 30C potencies, from which the patient will self-select. Many makers of these products will supply a simple key to help this process. Some of the most common remedies (e.g. Arnica for bruising or injury) are well-known best sellers and people keep them in their homes as part of a first aid kit. These are suitable for the non-specialist pharmacist to recommend with confidence; some are given in Table 3.2. There are several websites (e.g. those of Nelson's and Ainsworth; see further information list, p.241) which have an online 'remedy finder', where patients answer a number of questions about their symptoms and are recommended a remedy. The huge number of homeopathic remedies in use can cause practical problems for an average-sized pharmacy; usually a basic range is stocked and if necessary, manufacturers can normally supply a particular product by return of post (see suppliers list, p.139).

Dispensing

Apart from the commercially availably 6C and 30C potencies, pharmacists may encounter prescriptions for either higher dilutions or less common products, and there are some specialist homeopathic dispensaries which can make up individual remedies, using 'blank' tablets, hard and soft pills and granules, to which the potentized liquid is added dropwise. For dispensing homeopathic preparations, some form of training is needed and there are courses (notably by the Faculty of Homeopathy; see further information list, p.127) which provide instruction in more advanced aspects of homeopathic theory and also explain methods of dispensing. It should be noted that if dispensed on an FP10 prescription, homeopathic remedies attract an 'extemporaneous' dispensing fee.

How homeopathic remedies are taken

Tablets or pillules are released into the cap of the container and, without touching, are tipped into the mouth. They are sucked or chewed, and taken between meals. It is usually recommended that coffee, tea and other stimulants, strong-tasting foods and toothpastes are avoided when taking homeopathic remedies. The usual doses for adults and children are: two pillules every 2 hours for the first six doses, then four times daily for up to 5 days or until symptoms improve.

Evidence for the efficacy of homeopathy

The 'gold standard' for measuring clinical efficacy is the placebo-controlled clinical trial, where patients are given *the same drug* for the same condition. This is not compatible with the principles of homeopathy where an *individual remedy* is chosen for an individual patient, and for this reason the results of many clinical trials purporting to test the effectiveness of homeopathy are not accepted by homeopaths.

Various studies have given conflicting results but it seems to be the case that clinical trials of better (conventional) methodological quality tend to yield less positive results. This has not discouraged either homeopaths or patients and it has even been noted that negative publicity, for example in the form of television programmes, para-doxically *increases* interest in homeopathy. Dr Robert Mathie, research development adviser of the British Homeopathic Association, examined results from the best studies and found evidence that it works for eight conditions, including hay fever and flu, but has no effect on headaches, strokes or warts.

Occasionally, scientists attempt to find proof either that homeopathy works or that potentization and succussion produce measurable changes in the dilutions of the remedies. A few years ago, Jacques Benveniste published a paper claiming to show evidence for homeopathy in the journal *Nature*. However, subsequent investigation of his experimental methods came to the opposite conclusion, with a disastrous impact upon his career, and incidentally ensuring that only the bravest or most foolhardy scientist will venture into this area again.

In August 2005, *The Lancet* published the results of a study by Shang et al comparing the efficacy of homeopathy with conventional medicine. The study involved a comprehensive search for placebo-controlled trials of homeopathy up to August 2005. Nineteen electronic databases were searched, and 110 homeopathy trials and 110 matched conventional

135

medicine trials were analysed. In both groups, smaller trials and those of lower quality showed more beneficial treatment effects than larger and higher-quality trials. When the analysis was restricted to large trials of higher quality, there was weak evidence for a specific effect of homeopathic remedies but strong evidence for specific effects of conventional interventions. However, it was also emphasized in the paper that the trials examined exclusively addressed the narrow question of whether homeopathic remedies have specific effects. Context can influence the effects of any intervention, and the relationship between patient and carer might be an important pathway in mediating such effects. Thus for some people homeopathy could be another tool that complements conventional medicine, and future efforts should focus on the nature of these context effects to shed light on the place of homeopathy in healthcare systems.

Safety

Homeopathic remedies are generally harmless and suitable for everyone. There is a popular misconception that homeopathy is completely safe because it is 'natural'. This is not the case; homeopathy is safe because everything is very, very dilute. Since potencies above 12C are diluted beyond Avogadro's number, it is doubtful that a single molecule of the original starting material remains, so there is little potential for drug interaction or adverse events. Potencies at the lower end of the decimal and centesimal scales (up to about 3C) still contain measurable quantities of starting material and so theoretically may elicit pharmacological effects. These may be classified as prescription only in the UK; for example, Aconite (*Aconitum napellus*) 3C and 6X; Belladonna (*Atropa belladonna*) 2C and 3X; and Nux vomica (*Strychnos nux-vomica*) 3C and 6X.

There are isolated reports in the literature of suspected adverse effects, usually allergic reactions, following the use of homeopathic remedies. Many of the pills and tablets contain lactose (milk sugar), which may pose a problem for some patients with lactose intolerance. In such cases, liquid preparations can be given.

Homeopathic remedies for children

As homeopathic remedies are reportedly safe, many people use them for treating children. This is understandable at a time when conventional medicine is reluctant to recommend or even license many medicines for babies, because of fears of autism or other potential areas of litigation. Any of the appropriate homeopathic remedies can be used (see Table 3.2).

Homeopathic 'first aid'

A number of remedies have been deemed suitable for emergency use, in most types of patient (rather than taking a complicated symptom picture and prescribing individually). Examples of these remedies, including the well-known Arnica (for bruising and injuries), are given in Box 3.3.

External application of homeopathic preparations

Again, Arnica and Arnica cream are widely used to treat and prevent bruising after injuries, including accidents and surgery. In many cases, the products are not highly dilute, potentized preparations (although some are) but are more like herbal creams as regards concentrations. As this book is not a critical discussion of the subject, Table 3.3 is merely a guide to the products available and what they are generally used for.

References and Further Information

Kirkman M 2004 How does homeopathy work? Institute for Complementary Medicine. Available online at: www.i-c-m.org.uk/journal/2004/jan/005.htm

Shang A, Huwiler-Muntener K, Nartey L et al 2005 Are the clinical effects of homeopathy placebo effects? Comparative study of placebo-controlled trials of homeopathy and allopathy. Lancet 366:726-732.

Books

Dantas F, Rampes H 2000 Do homeopathic medicines provoke adverse effects? A systematic review. British Homeopathic Journal 89 (Suppl 1):S35–S38.

Ernst E, Hahn EG (eds) 1998 Homeopathy. A critical appraisal. Butterworth-Heinemann, Oxford.

Kayne S 1997 Homeopathic pharmacy. An introduction and handbook. Churchill Livingstone, Edinburgh.

Linde K, Scholz M, Ramirez G et al 1999 Impact of study quality on outcome in placebo-controlled trials of homeopathy. Journal of Clinical Epidemiology 52(7):631–636.

Booklets

From Nelson's: An introduction and guide to homeopathy; An introduction and guide to homeopathy for pets (see www.nelsonbach.com/en.html to order)

From Helios: Helios homeopathy: a basic guide to homeopathy (Aspinwall M) (see www.helios.co.uk)

Institutions and professional bodies

British Institute of Homeopathy Ltd

Cygnet House, Market Square, Staines, Middlesex TW18 4RH, England

Tel: 01784 440467 and 466251. Fax: 01784 449887. Email: britinsthom@compuserve.com Website: www.britinsthom.com

British School of Homeopathy

98a Mill Street, Torrington, Devon EX38 8AW

Tel: 01805 625494. Fax: 01805 625494. Email: learnhomeopathy@aol.com

Faculty of Homeopathy, The Royal London Homeopathic Hospital

Information on medical homeopathy for both the general public and statutorily registered healthcare professionals.

Website: www.trusthomeopathy.org

Society of Homeopaths

11 Brookfield, Duncan Close, Moulton Park, Northampton
    NN3 6WL
Website: www.homeopathy-soh.org
See also website information list.

Training courses in homeopathy

Hahnemann Academy of Homeopathy
The Registrar, 6 Livingstone Road, Gravesend, Kent DA12 5DZ
Tel: 01474 560336. Fax: 01474 327431. Email: info@the-hma.org
Department of Complementary Therapies
University of Westminster, Headquarters, 309 Regent Street,
    London W1B 2UW
Tel: 020 7911 5000
Website: www.wmin.ac.uk
Training courses especially for pharmacists
Faculty of Homeopathy
Dr Lee Kayne (Pharmacy Dean), 20 Main Street, Bushy,
    Glasgow G76 8DU
Tel: 0141 644 4344. Fax: 0141 644 5735
Manufacturers and suppliers
Ainsworth
36 New Cavendish Street, London W1G 8UF
Tel: 020 7935 5330. Fax: 020 7486 4313
Website: www.ainsworth.com
Nelsons Homeopathy and Bach Flower Remedies
Broadheath House, 83 Parkside, Wimbledon, London SW19
    5LP
Tel: 020 8780 4200 or 020 7629 3118 (specialist sales and mail
    order service)
Email: pharmacy@nelsonbach.com
 (Dublin: Tel: 00 353 1 679 0451. US: Tel: 001 978 988 3833)
Website: www.nelsonbach.com
Helios
Helios Homeopathic Pharmacy, 97 Camden Road, Tunbridge
    Wells, Kent TN1 2QR
Tel: 01892 536393 (24 hr) or 01892 537254 (9.45 am–5.30 pm).
    Fax: 01892 546850
Website: www.helios.co.uk
Weleda Ltd
Heanor Road, Ilkeston, Derbyshire DE7 8DR
Tel: 0115 944 8200
Website: www.weleda.co.uk

Table 3.1 Some popular homeopathic remedies suitable for pharmacist recommendation or patient self-selection: symptom picture and indications

Remedy, source and most frequently prescribed indication	Symptom picture	Better Worse
Aconite *Aconitum napellus* (plant: monkshood) Early stages of colds and flu; sudden onset of symptoms; fear and shock	High temperature with thirst; dry cough; great pain; bereavement; travel sickness; animal bites; anxiety; insomnia	In open or fresh air In a warm room or cold wind; late at night; with touch
Actea rac. *Actea racemosa* (plant: black cohosh) Depression, confusion, despondency	Depression; headache; stiff or painful neck/back; tinnitus; claustrophobia; heavy periods	When warm or when eating; headache improves in open air In cold and damp; when moving
Apis/Apis mel. *Apis mellifica* (insect: honey bee) Insect bites and stings	Burning, stinging pains; cystitis; swelling of lower eyelids; arthritis	Open air; application of cold Evening; heat
Argent. nit. *Argentum nitricum* (metal salt: silver nitrate) Fear of flying; fear of failure or of future events	Vertigo; tinnitus; colic; headache; dizziness from overwork; mental strain. Uncertainty and worry in irritable or nervous people	Open air; being occupied; walking fast Crowds; heat; sweet foods

Remedy	Symptoms	Better	Worse
Arnica *Arnica montana* (plant: arnica or 'mountain tobacco') Accidents, shock, bruising, exhaustion; after surgery	Injury, muscle ache; gout; sensitivity to pain; cannot bear touch; insomnia due to overtiredness; physical exhaustion; shock	Lying down; head lowered	Jarring movement; pressure on affected part
Arsen. alb./Arsenicum *Arsenicum album* (metal acid: arsenious acid; white arsenic) Food poisoning, with weakness, fear and thirst	Burning pains; dry throat; anxiety and fear; cramps and restlessness; psoriasis; aversion to food; desire for frequent sips of (usually warm) drinks	Warmth; lying down; cool air round head	After midnight, and around 1–2pm; cold wet weather; after cold drinks
Belladonna *Atropa belladonna* (plant: deadly nightshade) High fevers; delirium; flushed face; air sickness	Swollen joints; insomnia; facial neuralgia; throbbing headache; vertigo; colic; acne; cystitis	Lying down	Jarring movement; touch; mid-afternoon
Bryonia *Bryonia alba* (plant: white bryony) Dry, painful, violent cough	Dry mucous membranes; dry lips; great thirst for long periods; colds in chest; irritability; painful abdomen; colic; arthritis	Cold; cold foods and drinks; pressure (except on abdomen); rest	Any movement; heat; after 9 pm; eating beans or cabbage
Calc. carb. *Calcarea carbonica* (metal salt: calcium carbonate) Toothache; difficult teething; excessive appetite; premenstrual tension; period pains	Especially in shy, sensitive people; overweight; flabby; growth and developmental changes; poor digestion; craving for sweets or boiled eggs; fearful (e.g. dark, insects)	Dry weather	Teething; cold; wet; milk; heights; at night-time

142

Remedy, source and most frequently prescribed indication	Symptom picture	Better Worse
Calc. phos. *Calcarea phosphorica* (metal salt: calcium phosphate) Pain, especially after change in weather	Headache; period pain; rheumatic pain; fracture; injury where healing is slow; stomach pain after eating; grief	Warm dry weather; hot bath; rest Change in weather, especially cold and damp; exertion
Cantharis *Cantharis vesicatoria* (insect: cantharis beetle; 'Spanish fly') Intense pain of burns; cystitis; sunburn	Burning intense thirst made worse with cold drinks; intense mental and physical irritation; of sudden and violent onset	Warmth; lying down Cold drinks; coffee; passing urine; touch
Carbo veg. *Carbo vegetabilis* (plant origin: vegetable carbon) 'Rescuscitation' in collapse; lack of oxygen; digestive disorders	Sluggishness; cold body and breath; limpness and paleness; hoarseness; wind and bloated abdomen; overindulgence in food and drink	Cool air; burping or passing wind Warmth; fatty foods; tight clothing; dehydration; before sleeping
Chamomilla *Matricaria recutita* (plant: German or Hungarian chamomile) Teething children, especially with one red cheek	Intolerable pain, out of proportion to condition or injury; irritable children who cannot be placated, especially if hot and sweaty	Being uncovered 6–9 pm
Cuprum met. *Cuprum metallicum* (metal: copper) Cramps, especially abdominal with nausea	Nausea, vomiting; coughing with stomach cramps; cramps in fingers and toes; metallic taste in the mouth	After a cold drink; while sweating In cold air; evening and night; after vomiting

Drosera *Drosera rotundifolia* (plant: sundew) Whooping cough	Spasmodic, violent coughs leading to vomiting, retching or laryngitis; constant tickling cough	Open air; activity; getting out of bed Heat; warm drinks; lying down
Euphrasia *Euphrasia officinalis* (plant: eyebright) Watering, stinging or inflamed eyes	Cold with streaming nose and watering eyes; hayfever; conjunctivitis; inability to bear bright light	Dim light or darkness; cold compress Evening and night; warmth; indoors; bright lights
Ferr. phos. *Ferrum phosphoricum* (metal salt: iron phosphate) First stages of inflammatory diseases	Fever; colds; flushing; earache; nose bleeds; symptom onset slow and generalized; tired but alert; circular redness on cheeks	Exertion; standing up; cold; night-time Gentle movement; cold applications; warmth; summer
Gelsemium *Gelsemium sempervirens* (plant: Carolina or yellow jasmine or jessamine) Influenza; school phobia	Influenza; sneezing; heavy eyes; cough; sore throat; shivering; tired, aching muscles; prostration, especially in excitable and nervous people who have difficulty coping	Open air; after passing urine or while sweating Heat; sunshine; about 10 am; physical exertion; on receiving bad news; before thunderstorms
Graphites *Graphites* (mineral: graphite) Cracked, weeping unhealthy skin; eczema; dandruff	Impetigo; styes; dandruff; itching worse at night or when warm; encrusted areas; scabs; much oozing of sticky, honey-coloured fluid	At night; in warmth Cold

144

Remedy, source and most frequently prescribed indication	Symptom picture	Better Worse
Hepar sulph. *Hepar sulphuris* (metal salt or mineral: Hahnemann's calcium sulphide) Painful infected wounds; extreme coldness	Hypersensitivity to pain, touch, noise, exertion, cold; especially for the emotionally and physically sensitive or irritable	Warmth; heat applications; damp weather Cold; uncovering; pressure; night; dry weather
Hypericum *Hypericum perforatum* (plant: St John's wort) Injury to nerves after accident or wounding	Painful lacerations; falls injuring spine and coccyx; trapped fingers or toes; horsefly bites; bleeding piles; abscesses; tetanus	Bending head backwards Movement; pressure; coldness
Ignatia *Ignatia amara* (plant: St Ignatius bean) Acute emotional stress; bereavement	Acute loss, with shock and disbelief; prolonged grief, with sighing and insomnia, especially in sensitive and emotional people; croup	Warmth, eating Fresh air; suppressing emotion; coffee, alcohol, tobacco smoke
Ipecac. *Cephaelis ipecacuanha* (plant: ipecacuanha) Constant violent nausea; travel sickness	Nausea when vomiting gives no relief; sudden haemorrhage (piles, nosebleeds, periods); respiratory distress; bronchitis; salivation	Open air; resting with eyes closed Winter; dry weather; over-eating

Remedy	Indications	Better	Worse
Kali. bich. *Kalium bichromicum* (metal salt: potassium bichromate) Painful sinuses; colds characterized by thick, sticky and stringy mucus	Colds and sinusitis, especially after getting chilled; symptoms and pairs that come and go or move around; especially with listlessness and low spirits	Heat	Alcohol; very hot weather; mornings
Lachesis *Lachesis muta* (venom: bushmaster snake) Pain from sore throats, boils, abscesses, period pains; especially starting on left side	Pain and inflammation, especially in intense, jealous personalities ('volcanic'); symptoms much worse on waking, and start on left side of body; sensitivity to light and touch	Open air; cold drinks; during and after period	Sleep; waking; pressure; clothing; heat; sun; alcohol; menopause
Lycopodium *Lycopodium clavatum* (plant: clubmoss) Anxiety; lack of self-confidence	Fear of failure; irritability; hunger; craving sweet foods; bloating; flatulence; sore throat; earache; pains and other symptoms that start from the right side	Warm drinks; fresh air; activity	Stuffy rooms; loud noise; between 4 and 8 pm
Mercury Merc. sol./Merc. viv. *Mercurius solubilis* (mineral: Hahnemann's 'soluble mercury') *Mercurius vivus* (metal element: mercury 'quicksilver') Mouth ulcers; acute inflammation of skin and mucous membranes; acute sensitivity to temperature	Both remedies considered for the same indications. Inflammatory eye and ear and skin infections, such as herpes, and boils; with sensitivity to heat and cold; swollen glands; halitosis; excessive sweating and salivation, especially at night; thirst	Moderate temperature; resting; rising and sitting up; high altitudes	Night; open air and draughts; warm air and in bed at night; extremes of temperature and climate

Remedy, source and most frequently prescribed indication	Symptom picture	Better Worse
Nat. mur. *Natrum muriaticum* (salt: sodium chloride) Cold sores; mouth ulcers; acute inflammation of skin and mucus; silent grief, as in 'stiff upper lip'	Colds, sinusitis, runny nose, sneezing; eczema; thrush; urticaria; migraine; excessive use of salt on food. Oversensitivity, especially in patients who are insecure and irritable	Open air, bright light; cold water Mid-morning; seaside
Nux vom. *Strychnos nux vomica* (plant: nux vomica) Hangover; travel sickness; nervous indigestion; overindulgence	Digestive complaints; 'nerves', morning sickness or liverishness; stomach pain; constipation and piles after eating. Patients often work and play hard, with poor nutrition	Evenings; resting; warmth; being covered; after waking Between 3 and 4 am; cold, dry weather; draughts; anger; alcohol
Phosphorus *Phosphorus* (element: phosphorus) Burning heat and pains, especially in sensitive and volatile types	Bronchitis, cough and hoarseness, laryngitis and loss of voice; especially in impressionable people and those with a tendency to bleed easily. Heartburn	Open air; cold food and drinks; lying on right side Evenings; missing meals; warm food and drinks; sudden weather change; especially storms; lying on left side
Pulsatilla *Pulsatilla nigricans* (plant: Pasque flower) Childhood ear infections; catarrh and hayfever; menopausal symptoms in fair women; hangover; travel sickness	Changeable symptoms and patients; emotionally moody and tearful; craving company; clingy. Thick yellow or green mucus discharge; feverishness but lack of thirst	Open air; bathing; crying; cold applications; movement Cold, wet and windy weather; warm, stuffy rooms; hot food and drink; fatty food

Rhus tox.		
Rhus toxicodendron (plant: poison ivy)	Stiffness; restlessness; flu; colds; fevers; shingles; pains in joints and ligaments; tickly cough; tongue with red tip	Warm weather; heat; gentle continuous movement (after initial pain); rest; pressure
Sprains and strains; rheumatism; chicken pox		Prolonged rest; over-exertion; cold; damp; night
Ruta grav.		
Ruta graveolens (plant: rue)	Rheumatism; injury; bruising; eye strain; synovitis; urticaria; piles with prolapse of rectum	Movement
Injury to bone and tendon; sprains and fractures		Wet weather, cold; lying down
Sepia		
Sepia (mollusc: cuttlefish ink)	Hormonal changes; lack of energy; indifference and apathy; real and imaginary fears; sadness and loneliness	Warmth; exercise; open air; movement; pressure; hot applications
Hormonal and menopausal symptoms; depression		Pregnancy; menstruation; lack of food
Silica		
Silicea (mineral: silica)	Infections due to splinters, thorns; boils; constipation; acne; migraine and chronic headache; hayfever and sinus trouble, especially in pale and sensitive people; physical and mental debility	Summer; heat; lying down
Weakness; expulsion of foreign bodies: splinters, thorns, carbuncles, etc. (Not for patients with, e.g., grommets or metal pins)		Cold; damp; wet weather
Staphisagria		
Delphinium staphisagria (plant: stavesacre)	After surgery (especially childbirth) feels angry and resentful; does not like to be touched	Warmth; rest; breakfast
After episiotomy or other surgery		Exertion; missing a meal; tobacco

147

148

Remedy, source and most frequently prescribed indication	Symptom picture	Better Worse
Sulphur *Sulphur* (mineral element: sulphur) Skin complaints; itchiness; acne; piles	Skin diseases, especially with itching and burning. Aggravation from milk; liking for sweets; tendency to sweat; especially in intelligent sensitive types	Fresh air Warmth; bathing; warm drinks
Thuja *Thuja occidentalis* (plant: American cedar) Warts; styes	Warty growths and styes; pain and frequently passing urine; headache and lack of appetite in the morning	Flexion of limb; after sweating; massage Cold damp weather or direct sun; 3 pm and 3 am

Table 3.2 *Common complaints and homeopathic remedies to choose from*

Complaint	Remedies to choose from
Accidents, fractures, injuries and wounds	Generally: **Arnica** Before bone setting: **Arnica** Painful fractures: **Bryonia** After bone setting: **Calc. phos.** Bruises: **Arnica**
Acne	With red face: **Belladonna** Many pustules: **Hepar sulph.** In fair complexion: **Pulsatilla** With scarring: **Silica**
Anxiety	With fever: **Aconite** or **Arsen. alb.** With diarrhoea, fear or trembling: **Gelsemium** Anticipatory, with diarrhoea: **Argent. nit.** Anticipatory: **Lycopodium**
Appetite	Very variable: **Ferr. phos.** Loss of, with aversion to food: **Ignatia** Loss of, with cravings: **Arsen. alb** Excessive, feeling empty after a meal: **Calc. carb.** Hunger at night; easily satisfied: **Lycopodium**
Arthritis*	With swelling and redness: **Apis mel.** With bruised joints: **Arnica** With no relief from pain: **Bryonia** With variable, moving pain: **Pulsatilla**
Bad breath	With metallic taste in the mouth: **Merc. sol.**
Bereavement, grief	With sudden death, severe shock: **Aconite** Prolonged mourning, unable to get over loss: **Ignatia**
Bites and stings*	Red, hot, swollen: **Apis mel.** Animal, nerve pain: **Hypericum** Very painful to touch: **Staphisagria** Bluish around bite: **Lachesis**

Body odour	Profuse sweat, sticky, continuous, sensitive skin: **Hepar sulph.** Profuse sweating at night, chest, back and thighs: **Sepia** Sweat stains clothes yellow: **Merc. sol.** Unhealthy skin; worse in feet: **Sulphur** Sweating only on uncovered parts: **Thuja**
Boils, abscesses*	Small, numerous, sore: **Arnica** Burning: **Arsen. alb.** Hot, throbbing: **Belladonna** Slow to heal: **Silica** Itchy: **Sulphur** Painful, with pus: **Hepar sulph.**
Breast-feeding difficulties*	Engorged, hot, red: **Belladonna** Engorged, pale: **Bryonia** Abscessed: **Merc. sol.** Slow healing abscess: **Silica** Excessive milk: **Pulsatilla** Baby vomits or has colic: **Silica** Painful, with pus: **Hepar sulph.**
Bronchitis	With rattling mucus: **Ipecac.** With loss of voice or hoarseness: **Phosphorus**
Burns and scalds	With shock: **Arnica** If responsive to cold: **Cantharis** Deep, slow-healing burns: **Kali. bich.** *Externally: Arnica cream (unbroken skin)*
Chicken pox	Very itchy rash: **Rhus tox.** Feverish and fearful: **Aconite** Blisters containing pus: **Merc. sol.** With fever and throbbing head: **Belladonna** *Externally: Calendula cream*
Chilblains	Hot, itchy: **Pulsatilla** Inflamed, cold: **Rhus tox.**
Claustrophobia	With great fear: **Actea rac.**

Complaint	Remedies to choose from
Colds, flu	*See also Cough* Early stages: **Aconite** Watery discharge, cold: **Arsen. alb.** Watery eyes and streaming nose: **Euphrasia** Severe flu symptoms with shaking and prostration: **Gelsemium** Burning fever with chill: **Bryonia** Aching, restless: **Nux vom.** Thick, profuse discharge: **Pulsatilla** Thick, sticky, yellow discharge: **Kali. bich.** Sneezing, dripping nose: **Nat. mur.**
Cold sores	On lips: **Rhus tox.** Caused by sun: **Nat. mur.**
Colic	*See also Constipation* With fever and cramps: **Nux vom.** Better bent forwards: **Belladonna** Better with knees drawn up: **Bryonia**
Concentration (lack of)	Cannot concentrate: **Apis mel.**
Constipation	With thirst, headache: **Bryonia** With unproductive urging, or during pregnancy: **Nux vom.** Hard, knobbly stool: **Lycopodium** Small stools: **Nat. mur.** Large stool, painful straining: **Sulphur**
Cough, catarrh	*See also Colds, flu* After cold wind: **Aconite** Dry cough with chest pain: **Bryonia** Dry and night, looser in morning: **Pulsatilla** Croup: **Aconite** Croup on awakening, with sensation of a lump: **Lachesis**
Cramp	In calf muscles: **Arsen. alb.** Fingers, legs and toes: **Cuprum met.**
Cystitis*	Burning only when passing urine: **Apis mel.** Pain, and burning before, during and after urination: **Cantharis** Pain during and after urination: **Pulsatilla** After sex: **Staphisagria**

151

Dandruff	With scaling of the scalp: **Graphites** Moist scalp: **Sepia**
Dental treatment	*See also Teething problems* Fear of dentists: **Aconite** Before treatment (to reduce injury), bleeding gums, after-effects: **Arnica** Nerve pain after: **Hypericum** Symptoms after mercury fillings: **Merc. sol.**
Depression	Associated with despondency and confusion: **Actea rac.** Women who are easily depressed: **Sepia** In very emotional individuals: **Ignatia**
Diarrhoea and food poisoning	With vomiting: **Arsen. alb.** After eating meat: **Arsen. alb.** With anticipatory anxiety: **Gelsemium** Only on waking: **Sulphur** After eating fish: **Pulsatilla** After eating shellfish: **Lycopodium**
Earache*	From cold, with severe pain and fear: **Aconite** Stinging pain: **Apis mel.** Throbbing pain: **Belladonna** Windy weather, after swimming, unbearable pain: **Chamomilla** Ear red externally; after measles: **Pulsatilla** With discharge: **Hepar sulph.** or **Merc. sol.**
Eczema	Cracked, weeping skin: **Graphites** Dry, itching: **Sepia** Contact dermatitis: **Rhus tox** General rash, made worse by heat: **Sulphur**
Examination nerves	With diarrhoea or paralysis: **Gelsemium** With diarrhoea, feeling rushed: **Arg. nit.**
Exhaustion	After exertion: **Arnica**
Eye inflammation and infection*	From hayfever: **Euphrasia** Thick discharge, from cold: **Pulsatilla** Lids red and puffy: **Apis mel.** Watering, blocked tear duct: **Argent. nit.** Bruised: **Arnica** Eye strain: **Ruta**

Complaint	Remedies to choose from
Fear	Following an incident: **Aconite** To the point of terror: **Arsen. alb.** Of crowds, death, impending doom: **Ferr. phos.** Of darkness or thunderstorms: **Phosphorus** Of coming events (e.g. appearing before an audience): **Argent. nit.** Of failure: **Gelsemium**
Giddiness, vertigo	Looking up to, or down from, a height: **Argent. nit.** Rush of blood to the head: **Ferr. phos.**
Gout	With fear of being touched: **Arnica** With much pain: **Lycopodium**
Haemorrhoids (piles)	*See also Constipation* Very sensitive: **Hypericum** Pregnancy: **Nux vom.** Itching: **Nux vom.** Protruding, with much pain: **Ignatia** *External: apply Hamamelis*
Hangover	With sickness, nausea, headache: **Nux vom.** From beer: **Kali. bich.** From too much tobacco smoke: **Ignatia**
Headache	From chill, shock, fright; with sudden violent onset: **Aconite** Overexcitement or exertion: **Arsen. alb.** Throbbing headache; during period; from sun: **Belladonna** From change in the weather; with dry cough: **Bryonia** Violent pain at back of head: **Gelsemium** From grief: **Ignatia** Caused by sinuses: **Kali. bich.** With colds: **Merc. sol.** After rich food or loss of sleep: **Nux vom.** After ice cream: **Pulsatilla** After getting wet, or change in weather (damp): **Rhus tox.**
Hives (urticaria, allergic rashes)	With burning and stinging: **Apis mel.** With burning and itching: **Rhus tox.** After strenuous exercise: **Nat. mur.**

153

Jet-lag	For exhaustion: **Arnica**
	With paralysis: **Gelsemium**
Labour pains, childbirth	With fear of death: **Aconite**
	Intolerable pain: **Chamomilla**
	Weak, with back pain: **Gelsemium**
	Ineffective, with tearfulness: **Pulsatilla**
Laryngitis	With barking cough and dry throat: **Drosera**
	With hard dry cough and loss of voice: **Phosphorus**
Measles	Sudden onset, itchy rash: **Aconite**
	With eye inflammation: **Apis mel.** or **Pulsatilla**
	Bright red rash, hot skin: **Belladonna**
	Slow onset, dry cough: **Bryonia**
	Dark red face, headache, drowsy: **Gelsemium**
Menopause symptoms	Fair blue-eyed women: **Pulsatilla**
	Dark-haired women: **Sepia**
Menstrual problems (including premenstrual tension or syndrome)	Period, with headache: **Calc. phos.**
	Late, scanty period due to fright or chill: **Aconite**
	Hot, heavy blood loss: **Belladonna**
	Period: nausea and faintness with pain: **Nux vom.**
	Pain before period: **Lachesis**
	Period and PMT, with breast tenderness: **Calc. carb.**
	Period, and PMT, with depression: **Lycopodium**
	Period, and PMT, tearful, with breast pain: **Pulsatilla**
	PMT: constant nausea before period: **Ipecac.**
	PMT, sad and emotionally erratic: **Nat. mur.**
	PMT, moodiness: **Sepia**
	PMT, quarrelsome: **Nux vom.**
Mouth ulcers	Caused by burning from hot food: **Cantharis**
	Painful, with increased saliva, bad breath: **Merc. sol.**

Complaint	Remedies to choose from
Mumps	With fever, restlessness and anxiety: **Aconite** Fever, painful, swollen glands: **Belladonna** Enlarged glands worse on right side: **Merc. sol.** Enlarged glands worse on left side: **Rhus tox.** If breast or testicles involved: **Pulsatilla**
Nosebleeds	After shock or injury: **Arnica** With cough: **Ipecac.**
Postnatal care	*Mother:* In all cases to help recovery: **Arnica** Disturbed sleep, effects of medication: **Chamomilla** Pains from damage to perineum or coccyx: **Hypericum** After episiotomy: **Staphisagria** Profuse bleeding: **Ipecac., Phosphorus** *Baby: remedy can be taken by the mother if breastfeeding; if not, put under baby's tongue* Shock, after violent birth; retention of urine: **Aconite** Apparent asphyxia: **Carbo veg.** Blocked tear duct: **Silica**
Psoriasis	Intelligent, tidy patient: **Arsen. alb.** Cautious, indecisive patient: **Graphites** Oversensitive patient: **Hepar sulph.** Deep thinking, independent patient: **Sulphur**
Rheumatism	Mainly in back and neck: **Actea rac.** Mainly in back and limbs: **Apis mel.** With fear of being touched: **Arnica** Aggravated by movement: **Bryonia** Pain mainly in tendons and muscles: **Ruta grav.**
Sciatica	Worse in damp, cold weather and at night: **Rhus tox.**
Shingles	Especially if scalp affected: **Rhus tox.**

155

Sinusitis	Inflammation of frontal sinuses: **Merc. sol.** Blocked, worse in warm room: **Pulsatilla** Nose blocked, dry, sore: **Silica** Thick, sticky, yellow discharge: **Kali. bich.** With headache, worse on right side: **Lycopodium**
Sore throat	Dry, red, burning: **Aconite** Swollen, burning, stinging: **Apis mel.** Dry, hot, difficulty swallowing: **Belladonna** Dry throat and mouth: **Bryonia** Excess saliva and bad breath: **Merc. sol.**
Splinters	To ease out: **Silica**
Sunburn and sunstroke	Dry, red, throbbing skin: **Belladonna** Severe (take as soon as possible): **Cantharis** Made worse by movement: **Bryonia**
Teething problems	Red, hot cheeks with restlessness: **Aconite** Swollen, red, hot cheeks: **Belladonna** Red, hot cheek(s) with bad temper: **Chamomilla** Slow teething: **Silica**
Thirst*	With high temperature: **Aconite** For cold drinks: **Bryonia** Due to excess salt: **Nat. mur.** With dry mouth and throat: **Rhus tox.**
Toothache	Worse for cold air and drinks: **Calc. carb.** Better when cheek rubbed: **Merc. sol.**
Travel sickness	With restlessness and fear: **Aconite** With vomiting: **Ipecac.** Sensitivity to slightest motion: **Nux vom.** Airsickness: **Belladonna**
Vomiting, sickness	With diarrhoea: **Arsen. alb.** Caused by overindulgence: **Nux vom.** In babies: **Silica** Worse for coughing; with constant nausea: **Ipecac.**
Warts	Internally and externally: **Thuja**

* In these situations, a pharmacist may prefer to refer the patient to a GP if not already consulted, in case antibiotic or other treatment is needed urgently

Box 3.3: **A typical homeopathic first aid kit**

Contents
Aconite
Anti-bite tincture or cream
Arnica
Arnica ointment
Arsen. alb.
Calendula/Hypericum ointment
Gelsemium
Nux vomica
Rhus tox
Urtica ointment

The potencies commonly used in first aid are 6C or 30C.
Dosages: Follow the general rules for dosage. In first aid
work give doses often, hourly or 2-hourly for six doses. In
very severe cases every 10–15 minutes until better, usually
for 3–4 doses. **Source:** adapted from *First aid homeopathy in
accidents and ailments*, published by the British Homeopathic
Association.

157

1. **Bumps and bruises:** take *Arnica* tablets. Apply
   Arnica ointment. In any case of accident, take or give
   Arnica, frequent dosage in severe cases, say every
   10–15 minutes for four doses, less often for lesser
   severity.
2. **Bites and stings:** take *Aconite, Arnica.* Apply *Anti-
   bite* tincture. Additional remedies, *Apis, Belladonna.*
   Apis more particularly for bee and wasp stings, but
   also of value generally, if reaction severe with
   swelling and itching. *Belladonna* would be of use for
   heat and fiery redness with hard swelling and
   throbbing.
3. **Burns, sunburn:** take *Aconite.* Apply *Urtica* ointment.
   Serious burns must receive medical attention, but
   Arnica internally will counteract shock.
4. **Colds and chills:** take *Aconite.* If flu-like,
   Gelsemium. If hayfever-like, *Arsen. alb.* With gastric
   symptoms, *Nux vomica.* If there is a tendency for
   chestiness, have *Bryonia* with you.
5. **Cramp, from swimming:** take *Aconite* for chilliness.
   Nux vomica for spasm.

6. **Continental tummy, digestive upset:** take *Nux vomica*. For food poisoning, *Arsen. alb.*
7. **Heatstroke:** take *Aconite, Gelsemium* if lethargic and shaking. Additional remedy, *Belladonna.*
8. **Fracture:** take *Arnica*. Apply *Arnica* ointment.
9. **Sprains and strain, overexertion:** take *Rhus tox.* Alternate with *Arnica* if severe.
10. **Exposure to cold and wet:** take *Aconite.*
11. **Rescued from drowning:** take *Aconite* and *Arnica.*
12. **Grazes and cuts:** apply *Calendula/Hypericum* ointment. In any case of accident, shock, bruising, use *Arnica* internally.

Table 3.3 *Homeopathy: external applications*

External applications	Form	Indication
Arnica	Cream, tincture, lotion	Bruising, sprains, injury, muscular stiffness
Calendula	Cream, lotion	Bruises with skin broken Sore nipples from breast feeding Nappy rash Minor wounds and abrasions
Chamomile	Cream, teething granules	Toothache, sore nipples from breast feeding Nappy rash
Copper	Ointment	Cramps, muscular pains
Evening primrose	Cream	Sore, dry, skin
Graphites	Cream	Cracked, flaky, sore skin, psoriasis, eczema, dermatitis, dandruff
Hamamelis	Tincture, gel, cream, drops (often combined with calendula, horse chestnut)	Bleeding, piles, skin irritation, eye drops
Hypericum	Cream, tincture (often combined with calendula)	Wounds, abrasions, cuts, burns
Pyrethrum	Cream, spray	Insect bites, stings
Rhus tox.	Cream	Rheumatism, aches and pains
Ruta grav.	Cream, tincture	Sprains and strains
Tamus (black bryony)	Cream	Chilblains
Tea tree	Cream, gel, lotion, etc.	Antiseptic
Urtica urens	Lotion, spray (often combined with pyrethrum)	Insect bites, stings, itching, burns

Aromatherapy

Principles: the (usually external) application of aromatic oils to treat physical and psychological conditions

Positive aspects: often enhanced with therapeutic massage; suitable for palliative care and in the elderly and infants; little evidence of interaction with conventional drugs; pleasant, high patient acceptability; safe if appropriate oils, diluted with a 'carrier' oil, are used

Negative aspects: evidence for efficacy limited; may cause irritation or sensitization if certain oils are used; oils should rarely be used undiluted or taken externally

Development and general principles of aromatherapy

160

Aromatherapy, the topical use of essential (volatile) oils to provide therapeutic effects, is a very popular form of alternative medicine, with much overlap with the beauty and cosmetics industry, to the extent that much of what is sold as 'aromatherapy' is merely having a massage (or even bathing or showering) with fragrant oils. This has contributed to the view of aromatherapy as useless but harmless; however, it is increasingly being shown in clinical studies to have therapeutic benefits. The pharmacological properties of essential oils are well documented (Table 3.4) and it has now been demonstrated that essential oil components are absorbed through the skin and can be measured in the breath around 20 minutes after topical administration. However, it is not necessarily the case that topical application of essential oils mirrors exactly the effects of ingestion, since the different constituents may be differently absorbed.

Although it is often said that aromatherapy originated with the ancient Egyptians, there is no real evidence for this. The development of aromatherapy as we know it today is attributed to Rene-Maurice Gattefosse, a French perfumer and chemist, in 1928. Gattefosse is said to have burnt his hand while working in a laboratory and finding the lavender oil nearby, he plunged the injured hand into the flask. According to legend, the burn healed more quickly than would be expected, and with little scarring. During the Second World War, Jean Valnet pioneered Gattefosse's ideas using essential oils in wound healing, and progressed to using them more widely for other medical disorders. Marguerite Maury revived the traditional uses of essential oils for health and beauty and started the modern renaissance of aromatherapy, which has continued with the work of Robert Tisserand and others.

'Aromatherapy' is sometimes divided into three separate parts.

- **Aromatherapy** – the effect of essential oils on physical and psychological conditions
- **Aromachology** – the effect of aromas on emotions and feelings
- **Aromatology** – the internal use of essential oils, which can include vaginal or rectal administration as well as oral ingestion

---

Box 3.4: Summary of safety data for common essential oils

General points

- All essential oils shlould be diluted before use, with the possible exception of small applications directly to pimples or spots, or insect bites, of oils known to be safe in this manner (e.g. tea tree)
- Babies and children require even more dilute oils (see text)
- Oral administration is not recommended unless as 'waters' (e.g. dill water, peppermint water)

- All essential oils have the potential to cause sensitization or irritation in susceptible individuals
- Only oils known to be safe (see below) should be used in pregnancy; if necessary, consult a trained aromatherapist

Oils known to cause irritation or sensitization

Benzoin
Bergamot
Cinnamon bark and leaf
Clove
Laurel
Parsley
Pine (dwarf)
Rue
Sage (*Salvia officinalis*, not *S. lavandulaefolia*)
Savory
Taget
Thyme
Verbena

Oils to avoid in pregnancy

Bergamot
Camphor
Hyssop
Rosemary
Sage

Oils safe to use *externally* in pregnancy

Cardamom
Chamomile
Clary sage
Coriander seed
Geranium
Ginger
Jasmine
Lavender
Neroli
Patchouli
Petitgrain
Rose
Sandalwood

Table 3.4 *Pharmacological activities of selected essential oils*

Activity	Essential oil and plant species
Analgesia	Chamomile (esp. skin inflammation), *Matricaria recutita*
	Cinnamon (esp. oral and dental), *Cinnamomum* spp.
	Clove (esp. dental), *Eugenia caryophyllata (Syzygium aromaticum)*
	Eucalyptus (esp. rheumatic), *Eucalyptus* spp.
	Frankincense (= olibanum) (oral), *Boswellia serrata, B. carterii*
	Lavender, *Lavandula officinalis*
	Myrrh (esp. oral, mouth ulcers), *Commiphora myrrha*
	Neroli (= orange flower), *Citrus aurantium*
	Peppermint (esp. headache), *Mentha piperita*
	Petitgrain (from orange leaves and twigs), *Citrus aurantium*
	Pine, mainly *Pinus sylvestris*
	Sage (esp. oral, throat), *Salvia officinalis, S. lavandulaefolia*
	Thyme, *Thymus vulgaris*
	Wild thyme, *T. serpyllus*
	Wintergreen (esp. rheumatism, sports injury), *Gaultheria procumbens*
Antispasmodic	Anise (esp. colic, infants), *Pimpinella anisum*
	Basil, *Ocimum basilicum*
	Caraway (esp. colic, infants), *Carum carvi*
	Chamomile (German), *Matricaria recutita*
	Chamomile (Roman), *Chamaemelum nobile*
	Dill (esp. colic, infants), *Anethum graveolens*
	Fennel, *Foeniculum vulgare*
	Geranium, *Pelargonium* spp.
	Ginger (esp. colic, infants), *Zingiber officinalis*
	Jasmine, *Jasminum grandiflorum*
	Juniper berry, *Juniperus communis*
	Kanuka, *Kunzea ericoides*
	Lavender, *Lavandula officinalis*
	Lemon balm, *Melissa officinalis*
	Manuka, *Leptospermum scoparium*
	Marjoram, *Oregano marjorana*
	Peppermint, *Mentha piperita*
	Sage, *Salvia officinalis, S. lavandulaefolia*
	Spearmint, *Mentha spicata*
	Star anise (esp. colic, infants), *Illicium verum*

163

Activity	Essential oil and plant species
	Thyme, *Thymus vulgaris* Wild thyme, *T. serpyllus* Wormwood, *Artemisia absinthium*
Antiseptic, antibacterial, antifungal	Cinnamon (esp. oral and dental), *Cinnamomum zeylanicum, C. verum* Clove (esp. oral and dental), *Eugenia caryophyllata (= Syzygium aromaticum)* Eucalyptus, *Eucalyptus* spp. Geranium, *Geranium, Pelargonium* spp. Kanuka (= white tea tree), *Kunzea ericoides* Lemon balm, *Melissa officinalis* Manuka, *Leptospermum scoparium* Pine, *Pinus sylvestris* Tea tree, *Melaleuca alternifolia* Thyme, *Thymus vulgaris* Wild thyme, *T. serpyllus*
Anxiolytic	Bergamot, *Citrus aurantium* subsp. *bergamia* Clary sage, *Salvia sclarea* Jasmine, *Jasminum grandiflorum, J. officinale* Juniper berry, *Juniperus communis* Lavender, *Lavandula officinalis* Lemon, *Citrus limonum* Marjoram (sweet), *Oregano marjorana* Neroli (= orange flower), *Citrus aurantium* Patchouli, *Pogostemon cablin, P. patchouly* Rose, *Rosa damascena* Sandalwood, *Santalum album* Taget, *Tagetes minuta*
Cognitive and memory enhancement	Grapefruit, *Citrus paradisi* Rose, *Rosa damascena* Rosemary, *Rosmarinus officinalis* Sage, *Salvia officinalis, S. lavandulifolia*
Decongestant, expectorant and other respiratory	Benzoin, *Styrax benzoin* (Siam), *S. tonkinensis* (Sumatran) Cinnamon, *Cinnamomum zeylanicum, C. verum* Eucalyptus, *Eucalyptus* spp. Peppermint, *Mentha piperita* Pine, *Pinus* spp. Rosemary, *Rosmarinus officinalis* Sandalwood, *Santalum album* Tea tree, *Melaleuca alternifolia*

164

	Thyme, *Thymus vulgaris* Wild thyme, *T. serpyllus*
Hormonal problems, e.g. premenstrual syndrome, menopausal symptoms, dysmenorrhoea	Anise (esp. dysmenorrhoea, menopause), *Pimpinella anisum* Carrot seed (esp. PMS), *Daucus carota* Chamomile (German) (esp. dysmenorrhoea), *Matricaria recutita* Clary sage (esp. PMS, dysmenorrhoea), *Salvia sclarea* Dill (esp. amenorrhoea), *Anethum graveolens* Fennel (esp. dysmenorrhoea, menopause), *Foeniculum vulgare* Frankincense (= olibanum) (esp. dysmenorrhoea), *Boswellia serrata, B. carterii* Geranium (esp. PMS, menopause), *Geranium, Pelargonium* spp. Jasmine (esp. uterine disorders, childbirth), *Jasminum grandiflorum, J. officinale* Orange (sweet) (esp. PMS, menopause), *Citrus uurantium* (fruit rind) Rose (esp. PMS, dysmenorrhoea), *Rosa damascena* Patchouli (esp. PMS, dysmenorrhoea), *Pogostemon cablin, P. patchouli* Star anise (esp. dysmenorrhoea), *Illicium verum*
Insecticidal, insect repellent, insect bites	Cinnamon (esp. bites), *Cinnamomum zeylanicum, C. verum* Citronella, *Andropogon nardus, C. winteranus* Clove (esp. bites), *Eugenia caryophyllata (Syzygium aromaticum)* Eucalyptus (esp. repellent), *Eucalyptus* spp. Pine, *Pinus sylvestris* Tea tree (esp. headlice), *Melaleuca alternifolia* Thyme (esp. repellent), *Thymus vulgaris* Wild thyme (esp. repellent), *T. serpyllus*
Sedative	Cedarwood, *Juniperus* and *Cedrus* spp. Chamomile (German), *Matricaria recutita* Chamomile (Roman), *Chamaemelum nobile* Clary sage, *Salvia sclarea* Lavender, *Lavandula officinalis* Lemon balm, *Melissa officinalis* Neroli (= orange flower), *Citrus aurantium* Patchouli, *Pogostemon cablin, P. patchouly*

Activity	Essential oil and plant species
	Petitgrain (orange leaves and twigs), *Citrus aurantium*
	Rose, *Rosa damascena*
	Sandalwood, *Santalum album*
Stimulant	Clove, *Eugenia caryophyllata* (= *Syzygium aromaticum*)
	Eucalyptus, *Eucalyptus* spp.
	Hyssop, *Hyssopus officinalis*
	Peppermint, *Mentha piperita*
	Rosemary, *Rosmarinus officinalis*
	Sage, *Salvia officinalis*
	Spanish sage, *Salvia lavandulifolia*
	Tea tree, *Melaleuca alternifolia*
	Thyme, *Thymus vulgaris*
	Wild thyme, *Thymus serpyllus*
Wound healing and scarring, skin or hair conditioning, cleansing	Frankincense (= olibanum), *Boswellia serrata*, *B. carterii*
	Geranium, *Geranium, Pelargonium* spp.
	Lavender, *Lavandula officinalis*
	Myrrh, *Commiphora myrrha*
	Orange (sweet), *Citrus aurantium* (fruit rind)
	Pine, *Pinus sylvestris*
	Rose, *Rosa damascena*
	Rosemary (esp. hair), *Rosmarinus officinalis*
	Sage (esp. excessive perspiration), *Salvia officinalis, S. lavandulifolia*
	Tea tree (esp. infections, spots), *Melaleuca alternifolia*

NB: This list is not comprehensive and rarely supported by clinical evidence, but illustrates some of the most commonly used oils and their main applications in aromatherapy. Aromatherapists often make up their own favourite blends

166

Obviously there is considerable overlap (external application produces an aroma and also results in absorption) and therefore only the term 'aromatherapy' will be used here. The focus of this chapter is on the oils which are most commonly found in pharmacies, what they are normally used for, their therapeutic benefits (or otherwise) and contraindications.

Quality and safety of essential oils

Most essential oils are composed of up to 200 constituents, many of which are present in minor amounts, and of course, a minor component in one particular type of oil may be a major component in another, even from the same species of plant. Variation is commonplace even in natural oils and depends on chemotype, source, extraction method and storage. There is a great price difference according to quality, and this can lead to adulteration or falsification.

Natural products may have a different conformation (stereo-isomerism) and in the case of essential oils, 'optical' isomerism (chirality) is the most important. Chirality affects biological activity, since receptors are highly sensitive to the shape of a molecule. If the essential oil has been obtained from the correct natural source, chirality does not usually pose a problem but synthetically prepared terpenes often have the opposite chirality to the natural compounds and are more likely to cause allergenic reactions. If these are used to substitute or adulterate natural oils, the pharmacological and other properties can also be significantly changed and this is now considered to be a problem with some commercial products that contain essential oils.

Poor storage of essential oils leads to chemical degradation, oxidation and polymerization, which change the chemistry and hence the pharmacology. The available literature on this problem seems to show generally that it is a detrimental rather than beneficial change, particularly as regards irritancy. D-limonene of high purity is hardly allergenic at all, whereas d-limonene exposed to the air for 2 months sensitized guinea pigs when applied to the skin, due to an increase in the content of limonene oxide and hydroperoxide. Tea tree oil, which can actually reduce the inflammation induced by histamine in humans, can induce sensitization if allowed to oxidize to peroxides, epoxides and hydroperoxides. The odour of essential oils changes and the colour darkens as the oils degrade; this is a good indication of deterioration. It goes without saying therefore that only fresh essential oils, carefully stored in a cool dark place with the minimum exposure to air, must be used for aromatherapy.

Synergy and quenching

Synergy is the enhanced effect of a mixture, which is greater than would be expected from the effects of the individual components. For most purposes, it can be assumed that synergy is occurring when a more beneficial effect is obtained by a whole extract, or whole essential oil, than from isolated components. Synergy is normally assumed by aromatherapists to take place within oil from a single source, as well as in mixtures.

Quenching is a term usually applied to a reduction in sensitization or irritation caused by a major constituent which is quenched by the presence of the others. Two examples of quenching normally quoted are those of limonene, which can reduce the sensitizing potential of citral (both of which are found in most citrus oils), and eugenol, which can reduce the irritation of cinnamaldehyde (both found in cinnamon leaf oil). Further evidence is required for complete validation of the phenomenon of quenching.

Gender differences

Gender differences in susceptibility to drugs are now being investigated and apart from hormonal drugs, most examples relate to pain thresholds and responses to analgesics. It is known that there are gender differences in sensitivity to smell and the effect of odours on the brain, which is particularly relevant to aromatherapy. This science is in its infancy and as yet it is difficult to extrapolate further. However, it seems to be the case that women are more susceptible to the effect of odours and may therefore benefit more from aromatherapy, although at present this is pure speculation.

Route of administration of essential oils

Definitions of aromatherapy sometimes exclude the use of orally administered essential oils but oral ingestion is of course commonplace, due to the ubiquity of these oils in medicines, food and beverages. For gastrointestinal use as an antispasmodic, there is no real reason why peppermint, caraway, dill, fennel and similar oils should not be given orally *if well diluted and the dose carefully monitored.* When applied in the form of massage, the oils will be inhaled and will also stimulate the olfactory system with an aroma. Inhalation of an essential oil, perhaps in steam or otherwise, will lead to absorption into the bloodstream via the lung. This is not quite the same as olfaction (perception of an odour), which is possible with concentrations much too low to penetrate into the bloodstream.

The effects of odour are probably as important as systemic absorption, as odours can affect mood and other psychological parameters via the limbic system of the brain. Olfaction is an area where sex differences are important regarding pain perception and mood. Olfaction also elicits measurable physiological effects, such as the release of acetylcholine in rats by lemon oil. It is likely that the overall effect of an inhaled essential oil is the result of a combination of olfaction and its effect on perception and mood, and inhalation leading to therapeutically active blood levels. Inhalation is the method of choice for respiratory conditions as it delivers the essential oil directly to the oral mucosa and the airways but even then, topical application or chest rub may be used to ensure a longer term of action, as the warmth of the body volatilizes the oil over a period of time.

Suppositories, pessaries, tampons or douches can be used to deliver drugs via the rectum and vagina, either locally or systemically. They are not often used for essential oils but there is no reason why not, provided that the oils are well dispersed and diluted to avoid irritation to the delicate mucous membranes. Tea tree oil is often successfully applied locally for infections of the vagina.

Absorption through the skin is the usual method of administration in aromatherapy as it combines the therapeutic effects of the oils with the benefits of massage. Some inhalation will also occur naturally with topical application. The skin consists of several layers and it is known that components of essential oils, which are small lipophilic molecules, are passively absorbed in a fairly short period of time. Essential oils applied via the skin can be detected in the breath within 20 minutes of application, although the time taken depends on the particular oil. Application with heat, for example in a warm bath, can accelerate skin penetration. Some essential oil components are known to promote the penetration of conventional drugs through membranes and are used for this purpose in medicinal products such as ointments and skin applications, including dermal patches.

Formulation and application

Essential oils are always applied to the skin diluted with a 'carrier' oil, to minimize irritancy. One of the few exceptions to this is if, for example, undiluted tea tree oil is applied to skin eruptions. The carrier is a 'fixed oil' (as opposed to a 'volatile' or essential oil) such as almond, olive, peanut or other vegetable oil. Carrier oils may, however, not be completely inert and some are beneficial to the skin in their own right. They also make massage easier. Occlusion (covering a topical preparation with an impermeable skin) increases absorption even more.

As liquids, essential oils are normally measured by volume rather than weight; because these volumes are small, they are usually measured as 'drops' rather than in millilitres (ml). The relationship of drops to millilitres is generally accepted as **1 drop = 0.05 ml**; this will depend to some extent on the viscosity of the essential oil but is normally a good working definition. The carrier oil can be measured either way, depending on the volume required.

It is estimated that about 25 ml of diluted oil will be applied to the body during a full-body massage (Tisserand & Balacs 1995), so at a concentration of 4%, a dose equivalent of 1 ml pure essential oil will be applied to the body. Of this, up to 25% will be absorbed, giving a total *maximum* systemic dose of essential oil of 0.25 ml (= 5 drops). This is reasonable, and safe, unless an individual is allergic to a particular essential oil.

171

Non-medically qualified persons should not prescribe essential oils for internal use, although some carminative oils and decongestant oils are taken regularly in this way, often in warm water, such as peppermint or caraway oil for dyspepsia or eucalyptus or thyme oil for respiratory congestion. The oral dose is of the order of 0.5–1 ml or 10–20 drops, *over 24 hours,* which is considerably higher than that used in massage, even allowing for less than 100% absorption from the GI tract. This therefore demonstrates the relative safety of administering essential oil via dermal massage and inhalation, compared with the oral route.

Babies and children

Oral administration of essential oils to small babies is NOT recommended. Fatalities have been reported for such practices. If massage is required, more dilute preparations should be used as the skin of babies and small children is thinner and more sensitive. As a guide, a maximum concentration of 1% should be used for babies up to 6 months, 2% up to 24 months and after that, 3% until the age of 10 or 12, after which adult doses apply unless the child is very small for his or her age (Tisserand & Balacs 1995). Several products containing essential oils are now marketed for bathing infants and although these are safe because the oil is well dispersed or emulsified, it is usually suggested that drops of pure essential oils should not be added to the bath for babies less than 24 months old in case they are poorly dispersed and cause irritation.

Undiluted oils must never be instilled into the nostrils of children or adults, or applied to the skin as decongestants, and it is inadvisable to leave them anywhere near children who may accidentally spill or ingest the oil. Most instances of poisoning of children by essential oils are due to inappropriate use or careless storage.

Pregnancy

The use of some essential oils should be avoided during pregnancy, particularly during the first trimester. Although there is no real clinical evidence of safety, Tisserand & Balacs suggest that cardamom, chamomile, clary sage, coriander seed, geranium, ginger, jasmine, lavender, neroli, patchouli, petitgrain, rose and sandalwood can be used safely. Certain oils should definitely be avoided; for example, camphor, hyssop, parsley and sage. For others, caution should be exercised; none should be taken internally.

Epilepsy

The use of certain essential oils (those marked as 'stimulant' oils in Table 3.5) should also be avoided by patients with epilepsy.

Table 3.5 *Aromatherapy: Therapeutic indications for popular oils*

Oil	Common use
Anise, star anise	Muscle pain, menopause, dyspepsia, stress, exhaustion, water retention
Basil	Tonic, pain, nausea, stimulate blood flow
Benzoin	Inhalation for coughs and colds
Bergamot	Anxiety, depression
Carrot seed	Sedative, muscle pain, premenstrual syndrome
Chamomile (German)	Sedative, analgesic, antiinflammatory, dyspepsia, colic, premenstrual syndrome
Chamomile (Roman)	Sedative, analgesic, antiinflammatory
Cinnamon bark	Insect bites, sore throat, neuralgia
Cinnamon leaf	Analgesic, antiinflammatory
Citronella	Insect repellent
Clary sage	Depression, tension, PMS, menopause
Clove	Dental and oral pain, stimulant
Dill	Dyspepsia, colic, amenorrhoea
Eucalyptus	Insect repellent, insecticide, decongestant, expectorant
Fennel	Dyspepsia, colic, amenorrhoea, PMS, menopause
Frankincense (Olibanum)	Wounds, anxiety, stress
Hyssop	Stimulant, expectorant
Lavender	Sedative, hypnotic, analgesic, anxiolytic, stress, wound healing
Lemon	Sedative, carminative
Lemon balm	Sedative, hypnotic, analgesic, anxiolytic, antispasmodic, stress
Marjoram/oregano	Pain, headache, anxiety, depression
Myrrh	Toothache, mouth ulcers, skin problems
Neroli	Analgesic, anxiolytic, sedative

cont'd

Table 3.5 *Aromatherapy: Therapeutic indications for popular oils (cont'd)*

Oil	Common use
Orange, sweet	Skin conditions, hormonal problems
Patchouli	Sedative, anxiolytic
Peppermint	Carminative, analgesic in headache, stimulant
Petitgrain	Analgesic, anxiolytic, sedative
Pine	Insecticide, antiseptic, muscle pain
Rose	Anxiety, stress, PMS, memory enhancer
Rosemary	Stimulant, antiinflammatory, memory enhancer
Sage	Antiinflammatory, memory enhancer, sore throat, excessive perspiration
Sandalwood	Antidepressant, sedative, stress
Tea tree	Antiseptic, insecticidal, decongestant, expectorant
Thyme, wild thyme	Stimulant, insecticide, antiinflammatory, decongestant, expectorant

174

Drug interactions

None known or expected but some oils may enhance penetration of topical preparations.

References and Further reading

Clarke S 2002 Essential chemistry for safe aromatherapy. Churchill Livingstone, Edinburgh.

Lis-Balchin M 2006 Aromatherapy science. A guide for healthcare professionals. Pharmaceutical Press, London.

Tisserand R, Balacs T 1995 Essential oil safety. A guide for health professionals. Churchill Livingstone, Edinburgh.

CHAPTER 4

Physical therapies

INTRODUCTION

Pharmacists are much less likely to be involved with physical therapies but for patients in whom drug, herbal or other common therapies have failed or are either contraindicated or not acceptable to the patient, it may be appropriate to suggest a physical therapy. It is also common sense that if some form of musculoskeletal damage or misalignment has occurred, recourse to an osteopath or chiropractor is probably much more suitable than drug therapy.

In general, most of the therapies described below are safe and relaxing, with the obvious exceptions of manipulations which, if not carried out properly by an experienced practitioner, may dislocate joints (chiropractic, osteopathy), puncture the skin (acupuncture) or apply inappropriate pressure to damaged tissues (reflexology, massage, shiatsu). The only other concern is that, as with other forms of CAM, a proper diagnosis must be made and any serious illness treated in accordance with modern medical guidelines. This does not mean that CAM must be excluded but that it should ideally be viewed as 'complementary', rather than 'alternative'.

The most common forms of physical therapy are outlined in this section for information and so the pharmacist can advise the patient with confidence – whether to try or avoid! A brief definition and description are given below, with further detail available in the sections devoted to the individual therapy.

Acupuncture (from the Latin *acus,* needle, and *punctara,* puncture) is an ancient form of medicine which usually involves the use of fine needles to stimulate or unblock energy (Qi) flow around the body. It is commonly used in China, Japan and a range of Eastern countries and has recently become regarded as a valuable medical approach within Western medicine, where the numbers of medical practitioners and lay personnel training in this approach continue to grow. Related approaches include shiatsu (q.v.), electroacupuncture, acupressure and electrical point stimulation.

Chiropractic, from Greek *cheir* (meaning hand) and *praxis* (action), specializes in the diagnosis and treatment of mechanical disorders of joints and their effects on the nervous system. Chiropractic employs a technique of spinal manipulation based upon the theory that problems associated with vertebral alignment may result in neural, muscular or sensory disorders. Realignment of the spine aims to restore normal movement through manipulation. Related approaches include osteopathy (q.v.), spinal manipulation manual therapy (SMT) and physiotherapy.

Massage is the manipulation of body tissues using the hands, employing pressure and traction for therapeutic effect. It aims to enhance blood and lymph circulation by direct mechanical pressure and is effective for relaxation, premenstrual syndrome, anxiety and stress. Massage is usually a very safe technique, except in deep vein thrombosis, open wounds and osteoporosis, for example. Related approaches include Swedish massage, biodynamic massage, aromatherapy (q.v.), reflexology (q.v.), abdominal massage, sports massage and physiotherapy.

Naturopathy is a multidisciplinary approach founded on a belief in the power of the body to heal itself. Treatment is based on healthy diet, exercise, fresh air and water, but other natural therapies such as herbal medicine and massage may also be used. The term 'naturopathy' was first used in the 19th century and it is now practised in many continents.

Osteopathy is a system of manual medicine concerned with mechanical, functional and postural treatment. Therapy includes manipulation and palpation of joints, spinal vertebrae, muscles and tissues, aimed at resolving mechanical problems of the body. Osteopathy may be obtained in private practice and increasingly in the NHS. It is perceived as a well-established therapy, underpinned by extensive clinical training (4–5 years), which is central to the ability to make a differential diagnosis, in order to distinguish appropriate manual care. Associated therapies include massage (q.v.), manual therapy, spinal manipulation, chiropractic (q.v.), craniosacral therapy and posture-based therapies.

Reflexology employs varying degrees of pressure, commonly to the hands and feet, to promote health and well-being. It is based on the premise that the internal organs of the body are 'mapped out' on the surface of the hands, feet and ears. Treatment of internal organs is said to occur through gentle pressure to specific areas of the hands or feet, causing a therapeutic effect via 'reflexes or zones' that run throughout the body, terminating in the hands and feet. Similar approaches include massage (q.v), shiatsu (q.v.), reiki zone therapy, reflexology zone therapy, metamorphic technique, Morrell method, holistic multidimensional reflexology, Vacuflex reflexology.

Shiatsu, also known as acupressure, is based upon the same premise as acupuncture (q.v.) but rather than using fine needles to stimulate and harmonize Qi energy flow around the body, the practitioner applies direct pressure to key points (*tsubos*). Various applications using the principles of shiatsu are now commercially available, e.g. wristbands for the treatment and prevention of travel sickness, which have a metal stud incorporated to apply pressure at the relevant point; ear studs for insomnia, etc. Related approaches include: acupuncture (q.v.), moxibustion, reiki and massage (q.v.).

Acupuncture and acupressure

> **Principles:** involves the insertion of fine needles into specific points on the body to stimulate or unblock energy (Qi) flow around the body
>
> **Positive aspects:** suitable for use in conditions where drug therapy has been exhausted or may not work, for example in pain management, travel sickness, effects of chemotherapy, emotional distress, drug addiction and rehabilitation, the menopause
>
> **Negative aspects:** generally not advised in pregnancy, especially first trimester; bleeding disorders; pneumothorax; extreme emotional states; alcohol; strict asepsis required; preference for disposable needles (acupressure may be used instead)

General principles of acupuncture

Acupuncture is an ancient form of healthcare practice and medicine which aims to treat and prevent illness through the stimulation of the body's self-healing powers. It usually involves the use of fine needles to stimulate or unblock energy (Qi) flow around the body, together with herbs, diet, exercise and moxibustion, with the intention of restoring harmony and energy balance and therefore maintaining health. See also pages 45–46.

Underpinning this concept is a rich and complex theoretical system rooted in Confucian and Taoist philosophy that has been developed and refined over 2000 years through observation and clinical evaluation (Downey 2001). Acupuncture is commonly used in China, Japan and a range of Eastern countries and has recently become regarded as a valuable medical approach within Western medicine.

Acupuncture is one of the aspects of Traditional Chinese Medicine (TCM); others include herbal medicine, diet, massage and exercise. In Chinese philosophy the main organs of the body are linked to one of the Five Elements: Earth, Air, Wood, Fire and Water. These are said to form the circle of life (thus wood is burnt by fire and the ashes fall into the soil; earth creates metal that becomes molten with fire; water nourishes trees that in turn provide wood). This interlinked cycle is characteristic of many forms of alternative medicine and the integration of these approaches is based upon principles that all life is composed of energy. Thus the body is perceived as inseparable from the environment, a microcosm of the universe and permeated with the same energy (Downey 2001). In the human body this energy is dispersed through 12 main conceptual channels that are said to form an invisible matrix through which to convey and connect life energy. These are termed meridians, translated from the Chinese term *jing-luo* (*jing* meaning to 'go through' and *luo*, something that connects) (Kayne 2002).

Acupressure/shiatsu

Specific point pressure without use of needles is referred to as acupressure or shiatsu (see also Shiatsu, p. 211). This approach is popular with patients who are terrified of needles or for whom they are contraindicated (bleeding disorders). It also avoids the problems of maintaining asepsis and taking precautions against blood-borne diseases. However, due to the close proximity of certain acupuncture points, shiatsu may not be as accurate as acupuncture since more than one point may be pressed at any one time.

A particularly widespread application is the use of elasticated wristbands to reduce sensations of nausea. The wristbands have a 'button' attached which produces pressure at the wrist point P6. This particular point, which has been researched by Dundee and more recently by Schlager et al (1998), is suggested to reduce post-operative vomiting in children undergoing strabismus surgery. There is increasing research evidence to demonstrate reduction in nausea due to travel sickness, morning sickness during pregnancy and from the effects of chemotherapy.

Qi and the meridians

The energy described above is referred to as Qi or Ki (pronounced 'chee'). Qi is central to the day-to-day functioning of the body and continually flows through and around the organs. Health is maintained by a dynamic balance of two forms of body energy, termed yin and yang (see Fig. 2.1, p.47).

Imbalance or impedance of energy is said to result in a deficiency or blockage of energy, manifesting through symptoms and illness. Restoration of harmonious flow of Qi occurs through removal of energy blockage or treatment of energy depletion by accessing key points on the meridians. These are called acupuncture points or *tsubos*. More than 400 acupuncture points have been identified. These points can also be stimulated using heat from herbs such as mugwort, gentle direct pressure or the insertion of fine needles into precise points along a meridian line.

Whilst no direct evidence has been found to confirm the physical existence of meridians and their role in maintaining health, there is increasing evidence that stimulation of particular points does have an impact upon health and well-being.

There are suggestions that the position of certain acupuncture points corresponds with nerve pathways and that acupuncture stimulates certain neuro-transmitters such as serotonin and opioid peptides (Ernst 2001, Filshie & Cummings 1999, Han & Terenius 1982).

Box 4.1: Indications for acupuncture

- Back pain (Cummings 2001, Ernst & White 1998, Van Tulder et al 1999)
- Drug dependency (Avants et al 2000, Lipton et al 1994, Margolin & Avants 1999)
- Osteoarthritis
- Insomnia (Wang 1992)
- Nausea and vomiting (Schlager et al 1998, Vickers 1996)
- Migraine and headache (Vincent 1989)
- Weight loss and enhanced satiety (Ikezono et al 2005)
- Stroke (Ernst & White 1996, Gosman-Hedstroem et al 1998)
- GI disorders (Deihl 1999)
- Nausea and vomiting in pregnancy (O'Brien et al 1996, Smith et al 2003)
- Pregnancy and cervical ripening (Duke & Don 2005)
- Ear nose and throat conditions
- Cerebral activation (Bubnoff 2005, White et al 2004)
- Correction of breech presentation (Cardini & Huang 1998)
- Activation of the RB of neutrophils (Karst et al 2003)

Box 4.2: Contraindications to acupuncture

- Untrained use of needles – leading to bleeding and pneumothorax (Ernst 2001, Rampes & James 1995)
- Electrical stimulation of needles may be contraindicated with, e.g., implantable gastric stimulation (obesity treatment) or heart pacemakers
- Caution in pregnancy – though there are no absolute contraindications, moxibustion is not recommended and specific points should be avoided during first and second trimesters (Downey 2001, Ernst 2001). However, Smith et al (2003) conclude that acupuncture to treat nausea and vomiting in pregnancy is safe in the hands of a qualified practitioner
- Resterilized needles – infection

Diagnosis and treatment

A thorough history will be taken and tongue/pulse assessment may form part of TCM diagnosis.

The patient is asked to lie down and needles are inserted into specific points on the body. The patient may be left to rest with needles in situ for up to 30 minutes. The needles are then removed. The needles may also be warmed, stimulated electrically or vibrated. Patients may feel relaxed or tired after the acupuncture session.

Several treatments may be required but if the patient does not feel any improvement after 4–6 weekly or fortnightly visits, another therapy may be considered. Maintenance treatments at longer intervals may also be recommended.

References and Further Reading

Avants S, Margolin A, Holford T, Kostin T 2000 A randomised controlled trial of auricular acupuncture for cocaine dependence. Archives of Internal Medicine 160:2305–2312.

Bubnoff A 2005 Acupuncture activates the brain. Available online at: News@nature.com.

Cardini F, Huang W 1998 Moxibustion for correction of breech presentation: a randomised clinical trial. Journal of the American Medical Association 280(18):1580–1584.

Cummings M 2001 Acupuncture techniques should be treated logically and methologically. British Medical Journal 322:47.

Deihl D 1999 Acupuncture for gastrointestinal and hepatobiliary disorders. Journal of Alternative and Complementary Medicine 5.

Downey S 2001 Acupuncture. In: Rankin-Box D (ed) The nurse's handbook of complementary therapies. Baillière Tindall, Edinburgh.

Duke K, Don M 2005 Acupuncture use for pre-birth treatment. A literature review and audit-based research. Complementary Therapies in Clinical Practice 11(2):121–126.

Ernst E (ed) 2001 The desktop guide to complementary and alternative medicine: an evidence based approach. Mosby, Edinburgh.

Ernst E, Whie A 1996 Acupuncture as an adjuvant therapy in stroke rehabilitation. Wiener Medizinische Wochenschrift 146:556–558.

Ernst E, White A 1998 Acupuncture for back pain: a meta analysis of randomised controlled trials. Archives of Internal Medicine 158:2235–2241.

Filshie J, Cummings TM 1999 Western medical acupuncture. In: Ernst E, White A (eds) Acupuncture: a scientific appraisal. Butterworth Heinemann, Oxford.

Gosman-Hedstroem G, Cleeson L, Klingenstierna U et al 1998 Effects of acupuncture treatment on daily life activities and quality of life. Stroke 29:2100–2108.

Han J, Terenius L 1982 Neurochemical basis of acupuncture analgesia. Annual Review of Pharmacology and Toxicology 22:193–220.

Ikezono E, Takahashi G, Ikezono T 2005 Low caloric diet therapy with enhanced satiation by ear acupuncture and supplementary drink on an outpatient basis. New obesity research. Presented at 14th European Congress on Obesity, Athens, Greece.

Karst M, Scheinichen D, Rueckert T et al 2003 Effect of acupuncture on the neutrophil respiratory burst: a placebo-controlled single-blinded study. Complementary Therapies in Medicine 11(1):4–10.

Kayne SB 2002 Complementary therapies for pharmacists. Pharmaceutical Press, London.

Lipton DS, Brewington V, Smith M 1994 Acupuncture for crack cocaine detoxification: experimental evaluation of efficacy. Journal of Substance Abuse and Treatment II (3):205–215.

Margolin A, Avants SK 1999 Should cocaine abusing buprenorphine maintained patients receive auricular acupuncture? Findings from an acute effects study. Journal of Alternative and Complementary Medicine 5:567–574.

O'Brien B, Relyea MJ, Taeum T 1996 Efficacy of P6 acupuncture in the treatment of nausea and vomiting during pregnancy. American Journal of Obstetrics and Gynecology 174:708–715.

Rampes H, James R 1995 Complications of acupuncture. Acupuncture in Medicine 8:26–33.

Schlager A, Offer T, Baldissera I 1998 Laser stimulation of acupuncture point P6 reduces post-operative vomiting in

183

children undergoing strabismus surgery. British Journal of Anaesthesia 81(4):529–532.

Smith C, Crowther C, Beilby J 2003 Pregnancy outcome following women's participation in a randomised controlled trial to treat nausea and vomiting in pregnancy. Complementary Therapies in Medicine 10(2):78–83.

Van Tulder MW, Cherkin DC, Berman B et al 1999 The effectiveness of acupuncture in the management of acute and chronic low back pain. Spine 24:1113–1123.

Vickers AJ 1996 Can acupuncture have specific effects on health? A systematic review of acupuncture anti-emesis trials. Journal of the Royal Society of Medicine 89:303–311.

Vincent CA 1989 A controlled trial of the treatment of migraine by acupuncture. Clinical Journal of Pain 5:305–312.

Wang Y 1992 An observation on the therapeutic effect of acupuncture in treating 50 cases of insomnia. International Journal of Clinical Acupuncture 3(1):91–93.

White P, Lewith G, Prescott P, Conway J 2004 Acupuncture versus placebo for the treatment of chronic mechanical neck pain. A randomised controlled trial. Annals of Internal Medicine 141:911–920.

Chiropractic

Principles: chiropractic focuses upon the spine as central to the maintenance of health. Optimum neural balance is achieved by realignment of the spinal column through gentle manipulation

Positive aspects: suitable for back pain; low back pain; neck pain; migraine; tension headaches; some effectiveness with menstrual pain, colic and sports injuries. Cervical manipulation appears to be safer than NSAID complications in some cases

Negative aspects: avoid in advanced osteoporosis and arthritis, malignant spinal disease, severe inflammatory disease, patients on anticoagulation drugs or with traumatic injuries. Cervical manipulation and lumbar manipulation should only be performed by skilled practitioners

General principles of chiropractic

Chiropractic originates from Daniel Palmer (1842–1913) who manipulated the neck of a work colleague and allegedly cured his colleague's deafness. Palmer asserted that minor 'subluxations' (misalignments of the spine) could impact upon a person's health. Towards the end of the 19th century, Palmer developed a theory of musculoskeletal effects upon the central nervous system; this is based upon four premises, as shown in Box 4.3.

Ernst (2001) suggests that subluxation as the cause of all illness has no scientific rationale, although spinal manipulation has been shown to reduce muscular spasm and inhibition of nociceptive transmissions. There is, however, evidence to support short-term efficacy in low back pain, although Ernst & Assendelft (1998) note that some research on this topic is inconclusive (Cherkin et al 1998, Skargren & Oberg 1998). There is also evidence to suggest that chiropractic can have a positive benefit for

> Box 4.3: **The premises of chiropractic**
>
> - The body's inherent ability to heal itself
> - Centrality of the nervous system: 31 pairs of spinal nerves pass through openings in the vertebrae. If vertebrae are misaligned, this will cause pressure and inflammation, subsequently distort neural impulses and result in damage to surrounding tissue
> - Subluxation and joint misalignment interfere with optimal functioning of the neuromuscular system
> - Identification and treatment through manipulation of subluxations

non-migrainous headaches, but there continues to be a need for further research.

Some distinctions have been made between spinal manipulation therapy (SMT) and chiropractic, while other people use the term interchangeably (Kayne 2002). In the UK there are national guidelines on the treatment of low back pain, with Waddell et al (1996) noting that chiropractic manipulation is recommended as a symptomatic treatment for acute uncomplicated low back pain.

Diagnosis and treatment

- Thorough assessment of the spinal column is essential prior to any form of manipulation, using criteria summarized in the acronym PARTS.
- *Pain* – assessment of pain through percussion, observation, palpation
- *Asymmetry* – assessed using palpation, radiography and observation
- *Range of motion* – assessment of various types and range of motion
- *Tissue characteristics* – colour, tone, temperature, observation of swelling or abnormality
- *Special procedures* – ultrasound and other diagnostic procedures

Box 4.4: **Indications for chiropractic**

- Relief of low back pain
- Management of neck pain (Dabbs & Lauretti 1995)
- Relief of neck and back pain (Koes et al 1991)
- Migraine (Nelson & Bronford 1998)
- Neck dysfunction (Nilsson et al 1998)

Box 4.5: **Contraindications to chiropractic**

- Unskilled practitioner
- Advanced osteoporosis
- Malignant spinal disease
- Patients on anticoagulants (greater risk of cerebrovascular accidents)
- Mild initial discomfort
- Arteriosclerosis
- Traumatic injuries

Adjustment occurs through manual manipulation using parts of the hand and fingers. Direct and/or indirect pressure or thrust may be used. On average, patients should expect to need 4–6 sessions of chiropractic to feel the benefit.

Chiropractic and osteopathy are the only two complementary therapies regulated by statute.

References

Cherkin D, Deyo RA, Battie M, Street J, Barlow W 1998 A comparison of physical therapy, chiropractic manipulation and provision of an educational booklet for the treatment of patients with low back pain. New England Journal of Medicine 339:1021–1029.

Dabs V, Lauretti WJ 1995 A risk assessment of cervical manipulation vs. NSAID for the treatment of neck pain. Journal of Manipulative and Physiological Therapeutics 18:530–553.

Ernst E 2001 The desktop guide to complementary and alternative medicine: an evidence based approach. Mosby, Edinburgh.

Ernst E, Assendelft WJ 1998 Chiropractic for low back pain. British Medical Journal 317:160.

Kayne SB 2002 Complementary therapies for pharmacists. Pharmaceutical Press, London.

Koes BW, Assendelft WJ, Van Der Heijden J et al 1991 Spinal manipulation and mobilisation for back and neck pain: a blinded review. British Medical Journal 303:1298.

Nelson CF, Bronford G 1998 The efficacy of spinal manipulation, amitriptyline and the combination of both therapies for the prophylaxis of migraine headache. Journal of Manipulative and Physiological Therapeutics 21:511.

Nilsson NH, Christiansen HW, Hartvigsen J 1998 The effect of spinal manipulation in the treatment of cervico-genic headache. Journal of Manipulative and Physiological Therapeutics 18:435.

Skargren E, Oberg BE 1998 Predictive factors for the 1-year outcome of low back and neck pain in patients treated in primary care: comparison between the treatment strategies chiropractic and physiotherapy. Pain 77:201–207.

Waddell G, Feder G, McIntosh A et al 1996 Clinical guidelines for the management of acute low back pain: low back pain evidence review. Royal College of General Practitioners, London.

Massage

> *Principles:* the systematic, formalized manipulation of body tissues, primarily performed with the hands, employing pressure and traction for therapeutic effect
>
> *Positive aspects:* enhancement of blood and lymph circulation by direct mechanical pressure; effective for relaxation, premenstrual syndrome, anxiety and stress
>
> *Negative aspects:* avoid in deep vein thrombosis, skin infections, open wounds, osteoporosis; caution in pregnancy and beware reactions to specific oils (e.g. peanut oils to facilitate massage)

General principles of massage

Massage is one of the oldest forms of therapy, reputed to have been used by the Chinese in 3000 BC (Horrigan 2001, Kayne 2002). Hippocrates was said to have used friction for the treatment of a number of muscular disorders. The word 'massage' derives from Arabic, Greek, Hindi and French words associated with touch or pressing. Various techniques were refined by the Japanese and Middle Eastern cultures as part of their health and hygiene routines, although in Europe in the Middle Ages, religious dogma and superstition regarded anything related to physical or emotional pleasure as sinful. Not until the Renaissance did a renewed interest in aesthetics and health reinstate massage as a beneficial activity.

Many systems of massage are currently practised in the UK and elsewhere. For instance, Per Henrik Ling (1776–1839) developed a system combining exercise and massage to treat joint and muscular problems based upon the premise that vigorous massage could promote health and healing by enhancing circulation of blood and lymph. This approach was later termed

189

'Swedish massage' and introduced into the USA in the 19th century.

In 1870, massage was introduced to the United States from Europe; the first book on the subject was published in America in 1884. That same year, the Society of Trained Masseuses was formed in England, later to become the Chartered Society of Physiotherapists (1964). During both world wars, massage was used in the rehabilitation of injured men and in the early 20th century, nurses were trained in massage. However, the increased use of technology led to a decline in massage use by both nurses and physiotherapists.

More recently, massage has reemerged as a complementary therapy promoting a more gentle and calming approach, although in a number of European countries such as Germany, massage continues to form part of conventional medicine (Ernst & Failka 1994).

Many claims are made for the effects of massage. Some of these have been investigated and upheld by research and there is increasing evidence attesting to potential benefits of massage for a wide range of conditions such as musculoskeletal problems, back pain, water retention, soreness and fatigue, fibrositis, anxiety and depression, constipation, and even enhancement of the immune system. When performed by well-trained practitioners, massage techniques have a low risk of adverse effects. Pain relief is thought to occur due to the release of endorphins, also leading to relaxation (Kaada & Torsteinbo 1989).

Diagnosis and treatment

As with any intervention, massage must be planned following screening of the patient's medical history for identification of problems that massage may be able to relieve. The procedure should be explained to the patient and only undertaken after obtaining written consent. Practitioners may treat part or all of the body using direct hand massage with oil, essential oils or talc to facilitate the massage process.

The patient is made comfortable and covered with towels to expose only the part of the body being massaged, so that dignity and warmth are maintained at all times. Massage movements and gentle passive exercise of the muscles or joints are carried out in a logical order, according to the style of massage being used (see Box 4.6).

At the end of treatment, the patient is warmly covered, the therapist indicates that treatment is completed and the patient is left to rest.

Box 4.6: **The massage process**

Massage begins with slow, stroking movements (effleurage); this ensures a sense of calm and relaxation. The following movements are then used.

- *Tapotement* or percussion – striking surface of skin with side of hand
- *Petrissage* – kneading, squeezing and friction to loosen up tense muscles
- Friction and rubbing – slow circular movements to increase blood flow
- Vibration or shaking – to lower muscle tone
- *Effleurage* – deep stroking movements in the direction of venous flow. This improves circulation of surface blood vessels

Box 4.7: Indications for massage

- Relaxation for depressed adolescent mothers (Field et al 1992) and enhancing sleep in children (Ireland & Olsen 2000)
- Psychophysiological effects (back massage) for elderly institutionalized patients (Baldwin 1986, Fraser & Ross Kerr 1993)
- Emotional stress (Longworth 1982, Zeitlin et al 2000) and general reduction in anxiety levels (Field et al 1992, Fraser & Ross Kerr 1993)
- Anxiety reduction in child and adolescent psychiatric patients (Field et al 1992)
- Relief of muscular tension and fatigue (Balke et al 1989) and fibromyalgia (Bratteberg 1999)
- Premature and/or low birth weight infants (Vickers et al 1998)
- Improvement of local and distant lymphatic circulation (Mortimer 1990)
- Stimulation of local blood circulation, leading to a feeling of warmth (Hovind & Neilsen 1974, Kaada & Torsteinbo 1989)
- Low back pain (Ernst 1999a)
- After cardiac surgery (Stevensen 1994)
- Premenstrual symptoms (Hernandez-Reif et al 2000)
- Abdominal massage for chronic constipation (Ernst 1999b)
- Relaxation in AIDS patients (Birk et al 2000). NB: loss of weight and/or Kaposi's sarcoma may make massage uncomfortable unless gentle touch and extra lubricant are used
- Cancer patients – metastases are not caused or spread by gentle surface massage (Corbin 2005, McNamara 1993)

Box 4.8: **Contraindications to massage**

- Deep vein thrombosis
- Skin infections, burns or open wounds
- Advanced osteoporosis
- Extremes of body temperature
- Acute, undiagnosed back pain
- Fractures – direct massage
- Unexplained lumps and bumps – should be diagnosed before massage
- Unstable pregnancy – massage should not be given to the abdomen, legs and feet for the first trimester
- Chronic fatigue syndrome – patients may only tolerate short treatments when the syndrome is active
- Dementia and psychosis – such patients may be confused or frightened by massage and its effects

References and Further Reading

Adamson S 1996 Teaching baby massage to new parents. Complementary Therapies in Nursing and Midwifery 2:151–159.

Barr J, Taslitz N 1970 The influence of back massage on autonomic functions. Physical Therapy 50:1679–1691.

Baldwin LC 1986 The therapeutic use of touch with the elderly. Physical and Occupational Therapy in Geriatrics 4:45–50.

Balke B, Anthony J, Wyatt F 1989 The effects of massage treatment on exercise fatigue. Clinical Sports Medicine 1:189–196.

Beck M 1988 The theory and practice of therapeutic massage. Milady, New York.

Birk TJ, Mcgrady A, MacArthur RD, Khuder S 2000 The effects of massage therapy alone and in combination with other complementary therapies on immune system measures and quality of life in human immunodeficiency virus. Journal of Alternative and Complementary Medicine 6:405–414.

Bratteberg G 1999 Connective tissue massage in the treatment of fibromyalgia. European Journal of Pain 3:235–245.

Byass R 1999 Auditing complementary therapies in palliative care. Complementary Therapies in Nursing and Midwifery 5:51–60.

Corbin L 2005 Safety and efficacy of massage therapy for patients with cancer. Journal of Cancer Control 12(3):158–164.

Ernst E 1999a Massage therapy for low back pain: a systematic review. Journal of Pain and Symptom Management 17:65–69.

Ernst E 1999b Abdominal massage therapy for chronic constipation: a systematic review of controlled clinical trials. Forschende Komplementarmedizin und Klassische Naturheilkunde:149–151.

Ernst E, Failka V 1994 The clinical effectiveness of massage. Forschende Komplementarmedizin und Klassische Naturheilkunde 1:226–232.

Ferrel-Torry A, Glick O 1993 The use of therapeutic massage as a nursing intervention to modify anxiety and the perception of cancer pain. Cancer Nursing 16:93–101.

Field T, Morrow C, Valdeon C 1992 Masage reduces anxiety in child and adolescent psychiatric patients. Journal of the American Academy of Child and Adolescent Psychiatry 31:125–131.

Fraser J, Ross Kerr J 1993 Psychophysiological effects of back massage in elderly institutionalized patients. Journal of Advanced Nursing 18:238–245.

Grayon J, McKee N 1997 Massage therapy for patients with multiple sclerosis. International Journal of Alternative and Complementary Medicine July:27–28.

Hernandez-Reif M, Martinez A, Field T, Quintero O, Hart S, Burman I 2000 Premenstrual symptoms are relieved by massage therapy. Journal of Psychosomatic Obstetrics and Gynaecology 21:9–15.

Horrigan C 2001 Massage. In: Rankin-Box D (ed) The nurse's handbook of complementary therapies. Baillière Tindall, Edinburgh.

Hovind H, Neilsen S 1974 Effect of massage on blood flow in skeletal muscle. Scandinavian Journal of Rehabilitation Medicine 6:74–77.

Ireland M, Olsen M 2000 Massage therapy and therapeutic touch in children: state of the science. Alternative Therapies in Health and Medicine 6:54–63.

Kaada B, Torsteinbo O 1989 Increase of plasma beta endorphin levels in connective tissue massage. General Pharmacology 20:487–489.

Kayne SB 2002 Complementary therapies for pharmacists. Pharmaceutical Press, London.

Longworth J 1982 Psychophysiological effects of slow stroke massage in normotensive females. Advances in Nursing Science July:44–46.

McNamara P 1993 Massage for people with cancer. Wandsworth Cancer Support Centre, London.

Mortimer P 1990 The measurement of skin lymph flow by isotope clearance: reliability, reproducibility, injection dynamics and the effect of massage. Journal of Investigative Dermatology 95:677–681.

Porter SJ 1996 The use of massage for neonates requiring special care. Complementary Therapies in Nursing and Midwifery 2:93–95.

Reed BV, Held JM 1988 Effects of sequential connective tissue massage on the autonomic nervous system of middle aged and elderly adults. Physical Therapy 68:1231–1234.

Stevensen C 1994 The psychological effects of aromatherapy massage following cardiac surgery. Complementary Therapies in Medicine 2:27–35.

Vickers A, Ohlsson A, Lacey JB, Horsley A 1998 Massage therapy for premature and/or low birth weight infants to improve weight gain and/or decrease hospital length of stay. Cochrane Library. Update Software, Oxford.

Zeitlin D, Keller S, Shiflett S et al 2000 Immunological effects of massage therapy during academic stress. Journal of Psychosomatic Medicine 62:83–84.

Naturopathy

Principles: naturopathy is a multidisciplinary approach to healthcare founded on a belief in the power of the body to heal itself; treatment is based on healthy diet, exercise, fresh air and water

Positive aspects: since it incorporates a number of therapies, it can have broad potential and can also incorporate diet, massage, homeopathy, nutrition, hydrotherapy, detoxification and herbal medicine. Naturopaths are trained to refer patients with serious conditions for conventional treatment

Negative aspects: specific therapies in naturopathy, such as those involving excessive heat or cooling of the body, should be avoided in weak patients, during pregnancy, and in liver or kidney disorders

General principles of naturopathy

The basic principles of healthy nutrition, exercise and rest are well established as promoting health and well-being and are the foundations of naturopathy. The use of additional therapies can then be tailored to suit the individual's specific health concerns. Naturopathy can be traced back to ancient times and common ground is shared with systems such as Ayurveda and Traditional Chinese Medicine (TCM).

There are a number of systems of naturopathy practised around the world but they share a common philosophy, with the aim of maintaining health by supporting and stimulating the healing power of nature (*vis medicatrix naturae*) (Isbell 2001). All aspects of a patient are considered and treatment takes into account, for example, the physical type, diet, exercise, relaxation, massage and herbal remedies. Many of the principles of naturopathy are based upon the teachings of the Greek physician Hippocrates (c. 460–375 BC) who is considered to be the 'father of medicine' and who established the principle that practitioners should 'first do no harm' (*primum non nocere*). He maintained that health was dependent upon eating simple quality foods and exercising, and claimed that only nature heals and must be given the opportunity to do so.

According to naturopathic theory, disease occurs due to an imbalance in the body and this imbalance should be treated in accordance with natural laws. The cause of an illness should be identified (*tolle causam*), since symptoms are not the cause of disease but a response and reflect attempts by the body to purify itself via, for example, sweating, fever or diarrhoea and vomiting. Thus symptoms should not be suppressed as they are natural physiological mechanisms of detoxification. In Germany, *Heilpraktiker* (health physicians) are state licensed. Elsewhere, naturopaths are autonomous or self regulating (Isbell 2001).

Due to the eclectic nature of naturopathy, it may be necessary to refer to other chapters in this book covering other specific therapies.

197

Diagnosis and treatment

A thorough case history will be taken to identify symptomatology. At one end of the spectrum, there are practitioners who adhere closely to the 'nature cure' tradition, which focuses on diet detoxification and lifestyle advice. At the other end of the spectrum are eclectic practitioners who may use a wide range of therapies, including pharmaceutical-grade botanical medicines (Isbell 2001). Questions asked will involve general health and well-being, social circumstances, heredity and environmental factors. The precise nature of the therapy(s) offered will be contingent upon patient history and approach of the naturopath. However, naturopaths are trained to refer patients with serious conditions for conventional treatment (Ernst 2001).

The multidisciplinary nature of this approach can make it difficult to determine which facet of care 'catalysed' the healing processes of the body, and due to its complexity, only elements of this approach have been studied rather than naturopathy in its entirety. Any therapies incorporated within an individual's programme may need to be assessed independently.

Some therapies used in naturopathy

- *Chelation therapy* – this may also be considered a therapy in its own right and is a method for removing toxins and metabolic wastes from the bloodstream using, for example, intravenous ethylene diamine tetraacetic acid (EDTA) (Kayne 2002). The risks of chelation therapy outweigh the benefits and it has been suggested that this treatment should now be considered obsolete
- *Fasting and detoxification* – often with a herbal detoxification regime

Box 4.9: Safety considerations for naturopathy

- Naturopathy offers a wide range of therapeutic approaches; its safety, efficacy and cost-effectiveness have been well documented (Isbell 2001, Pizzorno & Murray 1999)
- Due to the basic premises underpinning naturopathy, other therapies are often only used after careful consideration
- The fundamental naturopathic tenets of diet, nutrition and exercise are employed in order to promote health synergy, but these are already well documented as being an integral part of maintaining health
- Contraindications to other therapies used as part of naturopathy should be referred to
- Excessive heating or cooling of the body should be avoided in weak patients, pregnancy, liver or kidney disorders (Kayne 2002)

- *Hydrotherapy* – bathing in hot hip baths; immersion baths; spa treatments
- *Enemas and colonic irrigation* – e.g. coffee or herbal enemas, to 'cleanse' the system and remove undigested food and 'toxins'
- *Hot or cold compresses* – to manage inflammatory conditions

References and Further Reading

Ernst E 2001 The desktop guide to complementary and alternative medicine: an evidence based approach. Mosby, Edinburgh.

Isbell B 2001 Naturopathy. In: Rankin-Box D (ed) The nurse's handbook of complementary therapies. Baillière Tindall, Edinburgh.

Kayne SB 2002 Complementary therapies for pharmacists. Pharmaceutical Press, London.

Pizzorno JE, Murray MT 1999 Textbook of natural medicine, vols I and II, 2nd edn. Churchill Livingstone, London.

Osteopathy

> **Principles:** a system of manual medicine concerned with mechanical, functional and postural treatment. Therapy includes manipulation and palpation of joints, spinal vertebrae, muscles and tissues aimed at resolving mechanical problems of the body
>
> **Positive aspects:** very effective for musculoskeletal problems; back and neck pain; intestinal problems and some respiratory disorders
>
> **Negative aspects:** avoid in osteoporosis, active bone disorders, brittle bone disease, spinal trauma, stroke, and direct treatment over infected areas

General principles of osteopathy

Osteopathy is a discrete clinical discipline involving mechanical, postural and functional assessment of the structure of the body and its relationship with problems affecting the neuro-musculoskeletal systems (Daniels 2001). Osteopathy emerged as a system of manual medicine in 1874 and the approach is still based upon the original three principles: first, that the body contains an inherent ability to combat disease and maintain health; second, that the structure and function of the body are interrelated; and finally, that the body is more than the sum of its parts: thus, dysfunction in the musculoskeletal system may contribute to other organ dysfunction such as constipation or headache. If the structure of the body is sound, the body is more able to maintain health and recover from illness.

Whilst there is evidence for the use of osteopathy manual therapy for the treatment of low back pain, relatively few research trials have been conducted objectively into treatment for other disorders. Osteopathic manipulation, used to treat musculoskeletal problems post surgery, was found to enhance mobility compared to control groups (Jarski et al 2000). Senior (1999) reported that at the end of a 12-week trial comparing medication treatment alone for low back pain to a regime including osteopathic treatment, there were no significant differences between treatment groups. However, whereas the group treated solely with medication was prescribed non-steroidal antiinflammatory drugs (NSAIDs) and muscle relaxants at levels of 54.3% and 25.1% respectively, those patients who also visited osteopaths were prescribed the same drugs at much lower levels, i.e. 24.3% and 6.3%.

As with a number of other therapies, there are also many case studies attesting to the efficacy of this approach. The General Osteopathic Council (GOC) reported up to a 40% improvement in symptoms of chronic fatigue syndrome following osteopathic treatment (GOC website: www.osteopath.org.uk/goc/links/research.shtml). Close links between chiropractic and osteopathy have resulted in research results conducted in one field being applied to the other.

Diagnosis and treatment

A treatment session usually lasts approximately 30 minutes, with 6–12 treatments constituting a full course. However, many people visit an osteopath on a regular basis to rectify any misalignment and prevent health problems developing.

A detailed patient history is taken, including mode of onset, extent, duration and severity of current or previous episodes. This may be categorized into congenital, developmental, traumatic, degenerative or pathological. Determination of pathological or psychosocial issues is also considered when assessing dysfunction. Examination consists of palpation to determine changes in tissue and muscle and observation of the body for posture and respiration, mobility and sensitivity. Passive palpatory examination is regarded as one of the hallmarks of osteopathy from which a segmental analysis is developed. X-rays may also be taken for further structural information.

Osteopaths do not treat conditions per se, prescribe medications or use invasive techniques such as injections. They work with their hands, using a wide variety of manual techniques including soft tissue stretching, passive movements to improve joint flexibility or high-velocity thrust techniques to improve mobility and joint movement (the audible click) (Daniels 2001).

Progress is monitored over subsequent treatments and therapy is perceived as a joint collaboration between therapist and client.

Craniosacral therapy

For certain conditions, particularly in babies and young children, craniosacral massage may be used. This involves gentle release techniques based upon the premise that cranial sutures have the ability to move very slightly. This manipulation is thought to enhance the circulation of cerebrospinal fluid, so relieving symptoms such as infantile colic, insomnia, irritability or certain behavioural problems. This should only be carried out by experienced and qualified therapists.

202

Box 4.10: **Indications for osteopathy**

- Low back pain (Andersson et al 1999, Assendelft et al 1995, Koes et al 1996, MacDonald 1988, 1990, Van Tulder et al 1997)
- Neck and shoulder pain
- Arthritis
- Headache
- Repetitive strain disorders
- Cranial osteopathy – infantile colic; behavioural problems (Holmes 1991, Vickers & Zollman 1999)

Box 4.11: **Precautions for osteopathy**

- Osteoporosis
- Spinal trauma after spinal manipulation
- Stroke following manipulation
- Treatment over neoplasms
- Infections

References and Further Reading

Andersson G, Lucentye T, Davies AM 1999 A comparison of osteopathic spinal manipulation with standard care for patients with low back pain. New England Journal of Medicine 341:1426–1431.

Assendelft WJ, Koes BW, Knipschild PG, Bouter LM 1995 The relationship between methodological quality and conclusions in reviews of spinal manipulation. Journal of the American Medical Association 274(24):1942–1948.

Daniels B 2001 Osteopathy. In: Rankin-Box D (ed) The nurse's handbook of complementary therapies. Baillière Tindall, London.

Holmes P 1991 Cranial osteopathy. Nursing Times 87:36–37.

Jarski R, Loniewski EG, Williams J et al 2000 The effectiveness of osteopathic manipulative treatment as complementary therapy following surgery: a prospective match-controlled outcome study. Alternative Therapies in Health and Medicine 6:77–91.

Koes BW, Assendelft WJ, van der Heijden GL, Bouter LM 1996 Spinal manipulation for low back pain. An updated systematic review of randomized clinical trials. Spine 21(24):2860–2871.

MacDonald RS 1988 Osteopathic diagnosis of low back pain. Manual Medicine 3:110–113.

MacDonald RS 1990 An open controlled assessment of osteopathic manipulation in non-specific low back pain. Spine 15:364–370.

Senior K 1999 Is osteopathy the best way to treat low back pain? Lancet 354:1705.

Van Tulder MW, Koes BW, Bouter LM 1997 Conservative treatment of acute and chronic non-specific low back pain. A systematic review of randomized controlled trials of the most common interventions. Spine 22(18):2128–2156.

Vickers A, Zollman C 1999 ABC of complementary medicine. The manipulative therapies: osteopathy and chiropractic. British Medical Journal 319:1176–1179.

Reflexology

Principle: based on the premise that the internal organs of the body are 'mapped out' on the surface of the hands, feet and ears. Treatment of internal organs is said to occur through gentle pressure to specific areas of the hands or feet, causing a therapeutic effect via 'reflexes or zones' that run throughout the body, terminating in the hands and feet

Positive aspects: safe; suitable when drug therapy not effective or contraindicated. Used for pain relief; relaxation; enhancing immune system; anxiety; migraine; constipation; labour management; induction of labour; premenstrual syndrome

Negative aspects: there is no known neurophysiological basis for connections between the hands, feet and internal organs. Direct pressure should be avoided over open wounds; some authorities suggest avoidance of reflexology in first trimester of pregnancy

General principles of reflexology

There is evidence to suggest that the therapeutic use of hand and foot pressure for pain relief and a range of symptoms existed in China and India over 5000 years ago. An image depicted on the tomb wall of Ankmahar, an Egyptian physician from 2300 BC, indicates that the Egyptians were familiar with hand and foot reflexology.

More recent developments of reflexology are commonly attributed to William Fitzgerald who was an ENT (ear, nose and throat) specialist at the end of the 19th century. Fitzgerald noted that gentle pressure to parts of the hand and foot could induce partial anaesthesia in areas of the nose and throat. In association with a colleague, Fitzgerald attempted to 'map out' areas or zones and in 1917 he published a treatise describing reflex zone therapy, suggesting there are 10 zones running through the body. He claimed that each zone manifested externally in the hands and feet so that gentle pressure on specific zones could produce a therapeutic response elsewhere in the body. He also claimed that, as with acupuncture or shiatsu, reflexology could stimulate not only the organ but also the interrelationship between organs and other body systems. In past decades this theory has been modified and adapted as therapists attempt to map the hands and feet, but differences in their approaches have resulted in a number of schools of reflexology.

Reflexology has grown in popularity over the past two decades and many claims have been made concerning its efficacy and value as a therapy. There appears to be a common consensus that foot and hand massage are efficacious in facilitating relaxation and thus provide some relief for stress-related symptoms. Reflexologists claim that pressure upon specific zones can facilitate specific symptom relief. There are also numerous case studies indicating the potential effects of reflexology (Coxon 1998, Tiran 1996, Wilson 1995), although such reports are much less robust than randomized controlled trial (RCT) data.

206

At present, there are few published RCTs to support claims (Poole 2002). In 1997 Siev-Ner et al conducted an RCT comparing the effects of reflexology with non-specific calf massage on 71 MS patients, using para-esthesiae, urinary symptoms, and muscle strength and spasticity as measurable outcomes. Significant improvements in urinary and spasticity symptoms were demonstrated, compared to controls. Oleson & Flocco (1993) investigated the use of reflexology for the relief of premenstrual symptoms, which resulted in statistically significant symptom improvement in the treatment as compared to the control group. Lafuente et al (1990) compared reflexology with the migraine medication Flunarizine; results indicated that reflexology was at least as effective as medication. A study by Launso et al (1999) also indicated headache relief following reflexology. Other studies conducted have been criticized for lack of sample size or scientific rigour and there is a need for greater research in this field.

More recently, Tiran & Chummun (2005) have discussed the physiological basis of reflexology and its use as a potential diagnostic tool. A number of studies have been undertaken to determine the extent to which reflexologists are able to diagnose (Baerheim et al 1998, Raz et al 2003), and Stone (2002) has also addressed the need for professional principles for reflexology practice. All conclude that further research is necessary.

Energy flow (Qi)

It has been suggested that when pressure is applied to reflexes, the natural energy flow of the body (Qi) is stimulated so that blockages, sometimes felt as gritty deposits under the skin, are dispersed, promoting harmonious energy flow around the body. The concept of channels of energy flowing around the body is not unique to reflexology and can also be found in acupuncture (q.v.) and shiatsu (q.v.). Dougans & Ellis (1992) have proposed that, like acupuncture, reflexology may similarly promote innate healing through Qi stimulation, but this issue continues to be debated.

207

Diagnosis and treatment

A full case history is usually taken by the practitioner. The patient may be sitting with feet elevated on a stool, or lying down. Hand or foot therapy usually follows a particular procedure, depending upon the style of reflexology employed. Each 'zone' will usually be treated systematically, employing direct pressure or massage. Painful or 'gritty' areas are identified and light to strong pressure applied. Oils may be used as lubricants to facilitate therapy. Treatment usually lasts between 30 and 45 minutes, and patients are encouraged to drink plenty of water following a session and to rest for a short while following treatment.

Some claims have been made concerning a 'healing crisis' involving posttreatment reports of flu-like symptoms, reduction in blood pressure, sleep or fatigue. These may be related to relaxation and whilst the 'healing crisis' is commonly referred to by therapists and has some anecdotal support, there is little research to substantiate these effects.

Box 4.12: Anecdotal and researched benefits of reflexology

Anecdotal benefits

- Reduction of stress-related symptoms: headaches, anxiety, insomnia and disturbed sleep patterns, and for general relaxation (Griffiths 2001)
- Labour and childbirth, for expectant and newly delivered mothers (Tiran 1996, 2002); retention of urine during pregnancy
- Symptoms of multiple sclerosis (Ashkenazi 1993)
- Reduction in hypertension (Trousdell 1996, Yongsheng & Ziaolian 1995)
- Relief of symptoms of back pain (Coxon 1998) and non-specified low back pain (Kovaks et al 1994)
- Infant colic (Wilson 1995)
- Heartburn and indigestion (Crane 1997)
- Nausea and vomiting

Researched benefits

- Relief of premenstrual symptoms (Oleson & Flocco 1993)
- Anxiety (Botting 1997)
- Relief of migraine

Box 4.13: **Contraindications to reflexology**

- Specific foot conditions such as gout; open foot ulcers; peripheral vascular disease
- Direct treatment over bony or soft tissue injury
- No clinical diagnosis should be made with reflexology
- Care should be taken when treating diabetic patients as foot injuries may be less well recognized in this client group
- Few other contraindications, but RCTs have shown no effect on asthma or on concentrations of serum cortisol during surgery (Engquist & Vibe-Hansen 1977)

References and Further Reading

Ashkenazi R 1993 Multidimensional reflexology. International Journal of Alternative and Complementary Medicine June:8–12.

Baerheim A, Algroy R, Skogedal KR, Stephansen R, Sandvik H 1998 Feet – a diagnostic tool? Tidsskr Nor Laegforen 118(5):53–55.

Botting D 1997 Review of the literature on the effectiveness of reflexology. Complementary Therapies in Nursing and Midwifery 3:123–130.

Coxon T 1998 Reflexology in the community. International Journal of Alternative and Complementary Medicine May:14–19.

Crane B 1997 Reflexology – the definitive practitioner's manual. Element, Shaftesbury, Dorset.

Dougans I, Ellis S 1992 The art of reflexology. Element, Shaftesbury, Dorset.

Engquist A, Vibe-Hansen H 1977 Zone therapy and plasma cortisol during surgical stress. Ugeskrift for Laeger 139: 460–462.

Griffiths P 2001 Reflexology. In: Rankin-Box D (ed) The nurse's handbook of complementary therapies. Baillière Tindall, London.

Kovaks FM, Abraira V, Lopez-Abente G, Pozo F 1994 Neuroreflexology intervention in the treatment of non-specified low back pain. In: Reflexology research report, 2nd edn. Association of Reflexologists, London.

Lafuente A, Noguera M, Puy C et al 1999 Effekt der reflexzone behandlung am fuss bezugliche der propylaktischen behandlung mit funarzin bei an cvephalea-kopschmerzen leidenden patienten. Erfahrungsheilkunde 39:713–715.

Launso L, Brendstrup E, Amberg S 1999 An exploratory study of reflexological treatment for headache. Alternative Therapies in Health and Medicine 5(3):57–65.

Oleson T, Flocco W 1993 Randomised controlled study of premenstrual symptoms treated with ear, hand and foot reflexology. Obstetrics and Gynaecology 82(6):906–911.

Poole H 2002 Researching reflexology. In: Mackereth P, Tiran D (eds) Clinical reflexology: a guide for health professionals. Churchill Livingstone, Edinburgh.

Raz I, Rosengarten Y, Carasso R 2003 Correlation study between conventional medical diagnosis and the diagnosis by reflexology (non-conventional). Harefuah 142 (8–9):600–605, 646.

Siev-Ner I, Gamus D, Lerner-Geva L et al 1997 Reflexology treatment relieves symptoms of multiple sclerosis: a randomized controlled study. Focus on Complementary Therapies 2: 196.

Stone J 2002 Identifying ethico-legal and professional principles in reflexology. Complementary Therapies in Nursing and Midwifery 8(4):217–221.

Tiran D 1996 The use of complementary therapies in midwifery practice: a focus on reflexology. Complementary Therapies in Nursing and Midwifery 2:32–37.

Tiran D 2002 Supporting women during pregnancy and childbirth. In: Mackereth P, Tiran D (eds) Clinical reflexology: a guide for health professionals. Churchill Livingstone, Edinburgh.

Tiran D, Chummun H 2005 The physiological basis of reflexology and its use as a potential diagnostic tool. Complementary Therapies in Clinical Practice 11:158–164.

Trousdell P 1996 Reflexology meets emotional needs. International Journal of Alternative and Complementary Therapy November:9–12.

Wilson A 1995 A case of feet. Australian College of Midwives Incorporated 8(1):17–18.

Yongsheng X, Xiaolian S 1995 Hypertension of pregnancy treated with foot reflexology – a case report. China Reflexology Symposium Report. Ankang City, Shaanxi: Foot Reflexology Service Centre: 68.

Shiatsu

> ***Principles:*** also known as acupressure, it is based upon the
> same premise as acupuncture (q.v.) but rather than using
> fine needles to stimulate and harmonize Qi energy flow
> around the body, the shiatsu practitioner applies direct
> pressure to key points (*tsubos*) to promote health and well-
> being
>
> ***Positive aspects:*** as with acupuncture, it can be an
> effective therapy for stress- and tension-related disorders,
> such as headaches and migraine, fatigue and anxiety;
> nausea and vomiting, including in pregnancy, motion
> sickness, postmyocardial infarction nausea and vomiting
> (PMINV) and due to chemotherapy; and also in
> constipation and period pain
>
> ***Negative aspects:*** avoid in osteoporosis, damage to the
> skin and underlying tissues (e.g. burns, bruises, wounds),
> varicose veins and in fevers

General principles of shiatsu

Shiatsu is also referred to as acupressure and uses
pressure points, as in acupuncture (q.v.) but without use
of needles. The term 'shiatsu' literally means 'finger
pressure' in Japanese but in reality the therapy is
performed with the use of pressure from fingers, hands,
elbows, knees and feet, along Qi energy pathways
known as meridian lines. It is therefore popular with
patients who are terrified of needles or for whom they
are contraindicated (bleeding disorders), and also
avoids the problems of assuring asepsis and taking
precautions against blood-borne diseases. At some
point in the history of shiatsu, there appears to have
been a schism which caused a divergence from its
Chinese origins and emergence as a Japanese therapy.
In shiatsu, the Qi energy of the practitioner is also
thought to have a beneficial effect upon the patient,
thus maintenance of health in the therapist is also seen

to be an influencing factor in treatment. The Chinese form of acupressure is referred to as *tui na*, in which a range of methods can be used, including rubbing and massage. The modern form of shiatsu was introduced to the West approximately 30 years ago (Gulliver et al 1993).

Much of the research conducted into acupuncture also has relevance to shiatsu. Harris (1997) and other proponents argue that there are differences between the positions of *tsubos* in shiatsu, and the number of meridian lines and their positioning appear to be slightly different in comparison with acupuncture. However, this is debatable. The most significant differences occur in the use of direct pressure rather than the insertion of needles into the body, the use of some aspects of massage and working with the patient's breathing patterns in order to gently extend or flex the body where appropriate.

Box 4.14: **Indications for shiatsu**

- General healthcare and to promote relaxation (Jarmey & Tschudin 1994)
- Tired eyes (Downer 1992, Stevensen 2001)
- Sinus congestion (Downer 1992)
- Menstrual cramps (Kayne 2002)
- Motion sickness (Bruce et al 1990, Hu et al 1995); reduction of nausea (Bayreuther et al 1994, Belluoumini et al 1994)
- Some digestive disorders; constipation (Stevensen 2001)
- Tension headaches (Stevensen 2001)
- Postmyocardial infarction nausea and vomiting (PMINV) (Dent et al 2003)
- Pregnancy and childbirth (see also Acupuncture)
- Pain and nausea relief in palliative care (Harris & Pooley 1998, Stevensen 1995)

Box 4.15: **Contraindications to shiatsu**

- Direct pressure on painful areas
- Osteoporosis
- Burns
- Broken skin and bruises
- Direct pressure over varicose veins
- Low platelet count
- Fevers, inflammation or swellings
- Skin infections

(Kayne 2002, Stevensen 2001)

Diagnosis and treatment

In shiatsu, visual, facial, tongue and *hara* diagnosis (gentle abdominal palpation) is performed prior to any physical treatment (Table 4.1). A detailed personal history will also be obtained. Between the weakest or 'empty' (*kyo*) and the strongest or 'fullest' (*jitsu*) meridian, a reaction is felt by the practitioner which can influence treatment (Stevensen 2001). Unlike massage, shiatsu is conducted with the patient wearing, ideally, loose cotton clothing. Therapy occurs over this with the patient initially lying down and then gently being moved according to the treatment required.

The approach employed can promote calm and relaxation. Points may also be stimulated using electro-acupuncture machines or by tapping on *tsubo* points.

A recent particularly widespread application of shiatsu or acupressure is the use of elasticated wristbands which have a 'button' attached to produce pressure at the relevant acupuncture point. These are used to treat travel sickness and morning sickness of pregnancy and many pharmacies sell them.

213

Table 4.1 *Examples of factors contributing to shiatsu diagnosis*

Time of day	5–10 am	10 am–3 pm	3–7 pm	7 pm–midnight	Midnight–5 am
Element	Wood	Fire	Earth	Metal	Water
Related organ	Liver/Gallbladder	Heart/Small Intestine	Stomach/Spleen	Large Intestine/Lung	Bladder/Kidney
Colour	Green	Red	Yellow	White	Blue/black
Sense organ	Eyes	Tongue	Mouth	Nose	Ears
Sense	Sight	Speech	Taste	Smell	Hearing
System	Nervous	Circulation	Lymph	Respiration/Waste	Renal/Hormone
Emotion	Anger	Joy	Reflection	Grief	Anxiety
Climate	Wind	Heat	Damp	Dry	Cold
Season	Spring	Summer	Late Summer	Autumn	Winter
Sound	Shouting	Laughing	Singing	Weeping	Groaning
Smell	Rancid	Scorched	Fragrant	Rotten	Putrid
Taste	Sour	Bitter	Sweet	Pungent	Salt

Adapted from Downer 1992

214

References and Further Reading

Bayreuther J, Lewith GT, Pickering R 1994 A double blind cross-over study to evaluate the effectiveness of acupressure at pericardium 6 (P6) in the treatment of early morning sickness. Complementary Therapies in Medicine 2:70–76.

Belluoumini J, Litt RC, Lee KA, Katz M 1994 Acupressure for nausea and vomiting in pregnancy; a randomised, blinded trial. Obstetrics and Gynecology 84:2456–2458.

Bruce DG, Golding JF, Hockenhulkl N, Pethybridge RJ 1990 Acupressure and motion sickness. Aviation, Space and Environmental Medicine 61:361–365.

Dent HE, Dewhurst N, Mills S, Willoughby M 2003 Continuous PC6 wristband acupressure for relief of nausea and vomiting associated with acute myocardial infarction: a partially randomised controlled trial. Complementary Therapies in Medicine 11(2):72–77.

Downer J 1992 Shiatsu. Hodder and Stoughton, Sevenoaks

Harris P 1997 Acupressure: a review of the literature. Complementary Therapies in Medicine 8:156–161.

Harris P, Pooley N 1998 What do Shiatsu practitioners treat? A nationwide survey. Complementary Therapies in Medicine 6(1):45–46.

Hu S, Stritzel R, Chandler A, Stern RM 1995 P6 acupressure reduces symptoms of vection induced motion sickness. Aviation, Space and Environmental Medicine 66:631–634.

Jarmey C, Tschudin V 1994 Shiatsu. In: Wells R, Tschudin V (eds) Wells' supportive therapies in health care. Baillière Tindall, London.

Kayne SB 2002 Complementary therapies for pharmacists. Pharmaceutical Press, London.

Stevensen C 1995 The role of Shiatsu in palliative care. Complementary Therapies in Nursing and Midwifery 1:51–58.

Stevensen C 2001 Shiatsu. In: Rankin-Box D (ed) The nurse's handbook of complementary therapies. Baillière Tindall, Edinburgh.

CHAPTER 5

Emotional and psychological therapies

INTRODUCTION

Emotional and psychological health is an important part of physical health, as shown by the placebo effect as well as by many other forms of complementary and alterative health systems. Of the various possibilities, pharmacists are only really likely to encounter the Bach Flower Remedies, which are sold in many pharmacies and health food stores. However, there is often an overlap between treatment modalities offered by homeopathy, aromatherapy and herbalism when treating emotional and psychological well-being.

The therapies listed in this section may be used in isolation or in combination and some therapies, for example, music therapy or laughter therapy, are so well embedded within daily life that it may seem unusual to list them here. Nevertheless, increasing research in this field is highlighting the impact of such therapies upon well-being. The list in this section is not exhaustive and is presented in order to provide a brief overview for both pharmacist and the people seeking advice. Where conventional drug therapy is contraindicated or not wanted by the patient, it may be appropriate to recommend one of the therapies listed below. Hypnotherapy is probably the most widely known therapy in this section and it is commonly used for the treatment of addictions to tobacco and narcotics, for example, and also for stress, phobias and insomnia.

Bach Flower Remedies were created in the 1930s by Edward Bach, a Harley Street doctor, who considered that the true cause of illness in human beings lies in the personality and emotional well-being. Although Bach Flower Remedies offer little, if any, scientific evidence of efficacy, they are very popular and widely sold in pharmacies. The most commonly used remedy is 'Rescue Remedy' which is promoted for use in times of emotional crisis.

Healing is a form of energy exchange between the healer and patient, which can result in a subsequent improvement in symptoms and well-being. The term is also used generically to describe specific 'healing' practices. Related techniques include therapeutic touch, non-contact touch, spiritual healing, lying on of hands, meditation and reiki.

Hypnotherapy is the deliberate use of the trance state to effect change in the conscious (e.g. breathing) and/or the autonomic nervous system (gut peristalsis, blood pressure). The individual, *not* the therapist, is considered to be in control of their trance state. Thus hypnosis is fundamentally self-hypnosis with the therapist acting as a facilitator. Related techniques include visualization, biofeedback and meditation.

Music therapy has many physiological and psycho-logical benefits. It is a common complementary therapy treatment in North American hospitals where trials have shown it is effective in reducing pain and anxiety. However, the choice of music is important and evidence suggests that some forms of music are aggressive, and violent lyrics may have negative effects upon an individual. Related therapies include dance therapy, singing, music as therapy, relaxation and pain management.

Bach Flower Remedies

> **Principles:** non-scientific, 'emotional therapy'; placebo effect likely to be high. Each flower remedy is supposed to aid a specific emotion, providing a 'correcting vibration' for a state of mind that needs to be 'rebalanced'
>
> **Positive aspects:** suitable for pregnant women and children; no drug interactions, no adverse drug reactions
>
> **Negative aspects:** no evidence of efficacy; no pharmacological or clinical studies

General principles of Bach Flower Remedies

The Bach Flower Remedies are 38 plant- and flower-based remedies created in the 1930s by Dr Edward Bach, a Harley Street doctor, who considered that the true cause of human illness lies in the personality, and developed the remedies to help people manage the emotional demands of everyday life. They are produced by steeping the chosen flower species in spring or spa water and preserving with brandy, and can be taken individually or mixed together to match the way the patient feels (see Table 5.1).

Although their proposed action is not consistent with scientific medicine as viewed by pharmacists or doctors, Bach Flower Remedies are very popular, especially the 'Rescue Remedy' which is a sort of first aid kit in a bottle, used in times of emotional crisis. According to the Bach Centre, there are no contraindications and no side effects. The drops do, however, contain alcohol, although in small amounts. There are virtually no objective RCT studies to support claims.

Rescue Remedy (an 'emergency' combination containing five flower remedies: Impatiens, Star of Bethlehem, Cherry Plum, Rock Rose and Clematis) in particular appears to be very much in favour with celebrities and

219

actors for stress or stage fright but on a more mundane level, some parents find it useful for children, who may not actually need any analgesic or other medication (e.g. after a minor fall) but respond well (i.e. stop crying) after being given 'medicine'.

Table 5.2 gives the indications for each remedy; this is not an endorsement but an attempt to give a concise guide to aid self-selection *by the patient*, since this is the most likely scenario and some pharmacists consider it unethical to recommend non-scientific therapies even for their placebo properties. In general, most pharmacies stock the Rescue Remedy, which comes in two forms: drops for internal use (as with the other single flower remedies) and a cream for topical use. Health food stores

220

Table 5.1 *Bach's classification of emotional states and appropriate remedies*

Emotional state	Remedies
Fear	Aspen, Cherry Plum, Mimulus, Red Chestnut, Rock Rose
Loneliness	Heather, Impatients, Water Violet
Uncertainty	Cerato, Gentian, Gorse, Hornbeam, Scleranthus, Wild Oat
Lack of interest	Chestnut Bud, Clematis, Honeysuckle, Mustard, Olive, Wild Rose, White Chestnut
Despondency and despair	Crab Apple, Elm, Larch, Oak, Pine, Star of Bethlehem, Sweet Chestnut, Willow
Oversensitivity	Agrimony, Centaury, Holly, Walnut
Overconcern for others	Beech, Chicory, Rock Water, Vervain, Vine
Rescue Remedy drops: for panic attacks, emotional crises, acute distress, sudden shock. *Rescue Remedy cream: for sore or injured skin*	A combination of Impatiens, Star of Bethlehem, Cherry Plum, Rock Rose and Clematis

Table 5.2 *Specific flower remedy and indicated emotional state*

Flower remedy	Emotional state
Agrimony	Mental torment hidden behind a mask
Aspen	Fear of the unknown
Beech	Lack of tolerance or coming to terms with life
Centaury	Difficulty in refusing requests from others
Cerato	Lack of confidence in one's own judgement
Cherry Plum	Fear of mental weakness or breakdown
Chestnut Bud	Failure to learn from mistakes
Chicory	Possessive, selfish love
Clematis	Procrastination with lack of focus
Crab Apple	The cleansing remedy; also for self-loathing
Elm	Overwhelmed by responsibilities
Gentian	Despondency, especially after a setback
Gorse	Hopelessness and despair
Heather	Self-centredness
Holly	Envy, jealousy, hatred
Honeysuckle	Living in the past
Hornbeam	Procrastination with tiredness
Impatiens	Impatience
Larch	Timidity and lack of confidence
Mimulus	Fear of known things or forthcoming events
Mustard	Deep melancholy for no reason (depression)
Oak	Exhaustion from overwork and the inability to stop
Olive	Exhaustion following mental or physical effort
Pine	Guilt and remorse
Red Chestnut	Excessive worry over loved ones
Rock Rose	Terror and fright
Rock Water	Self-denial, rigidity and self-repression
Scleranthus	Inability to choose between alternatives
Star of Bethlehem	Shock

221

Sweet Chestnut	*Extreme mental anguish and despair*
Vervain	*Overenthusiasm followed by disappointment*
Vine	*Dominance and intransigence*
Walnut	*Fear of change or the unknown*
Water Violet	*Pride or superciliousness*
White Chestnut	*Unwanted negative thoughts and mental arguments*
Wild Oat	*Uncertainty over direction in life or future*
Wild Rose	*Resignation and apathy*
Willow	*Self-pity and resentment*

will usually stock the whole range. A complete kit is also available for those wishing to act as 'practitioners', often after undergoing a short online or correspondence course.

How flower remedies are taken

Remedies come as a liquid. Commonly, two drops are diluted with mineral water into a 30 ml dropper bottle and four drops are taken four times a day. Alternatively, two drops can be put into a glass of water and sips taken at intervals.

Any of the Bach Flower Remedies can be combined to make an individual treatment, to a maximum of six or seven. To make a combination, two drops of each essence are put into a clean glass dropper bottle containing up to 30 ml of spring or spa water, adding a teaspoonful of brandy or cider vinegar as a preservative.

The length of time taken to see an improvement depends on many factors, including how long the patient has remained in the negative state and their sensitivity. It is usually recommended that adults should take their chosen selection for 6–8 weeks (for long-standing problems) and then review to see which essences have worked or if any new or underlying states have appeared, and continue to treat these. For relief from very recent or immediate negative states, and for Rescue Remedy, put two drops of each essence in a drink and sip or, if diluting liquid is unavailable, two drops from the stock bottle straight onto the tongue and repeat as needed.

Selection of flower remedy

The remedies are intended to be so simple to use that anyone could select and take them without professional advice or the need for any special techniques, and the Bach Centre gives some examples on its website (www.bachcentre.com).

Edward Bach divided his flower remedies into seven different groups (plus Rescue Remedy), each group representing a particular mental or emotional state. These groups, together with the recommended remedies, are shown in Table 5.1. The individual characteristics of each remedy are given in Table 5.2.

Further reading and Further information

Dr Edward Bach Foundation, Bach Centre, Mount Vernon, Bakers Lane, Sotwell, Oxon, OX10 0PZ, UK.
Tel: +44 (0) 1491 834678. Fax: +44 (0) 1491 825022
Website: www.bachcentre.com
Weeks S, Bullen V 1973 Bach Flower Remedies: illustrations and preparations, 2nd edn. C W Daniels, London, UK.

Healing

Principles: therapeutic form of energy exchange based upon a cause-and-effect relationship between conscious intention of the healer to heal, with a subsequent improvement in client symptoms and physical and psychological well-being

Positive aspects: safe; may give comfort in difficult or terminal situations; can be used in concordance with religious beliefs. Used for pain management; non-specific symptom relief; phobias, general maintenance of health and well-being

Negative aspects: intentional healing may be contrary to the client's world-view or religion, and this should be acknowledged

General principles of healing

Healing is part of the indigenous approach underpinning all forms of complementary therapy, although it may also be perceived as a specific therapeutic modality. There are various approaches to healing, e.g. spiritual healing, shamanism, reiki (see Box 5.1) and these are influenced by the process, procedure and philosophical and epistemological framework adopted.

There is a growing body of literature addressing the ancient origins of healing and healing belief systems (Benor 1990, 2004, Glik 1990, Rankin-Box 2001). There are many forms of healing, and Benor (2004) describes healing as 'any purposeful intervention by one or more persons wishing to help another living being to change for the better, using processes of focused intention, light manual contact or hand movements near the subject of the healing'.

Traditional indigenous healing is widely used across a range of cultures today (Struthers et al 2004). In January 2000, the National Center for Complementary and Alternative Medicine (NCCAM) announced a programme to support developmental studies to establish the methodological feasibility and strengthen the scientific rationale for proceeding to full-scale research clinical trials on the use of traditional, indigenous systems of medicine as practised in the United States (NCCAM 2002, Struthers et al 2004).

Spiritual healing can be traced back to the Koran, the Bible and the Torah. Shamanism seems to be at least 30,000 years old and can be found in almost all human cultures; it may be one of the earliest characteristically human activities influencing all human societies and belief systems (Money 2001). Shamanism represents a spiritual tradition incorporating a powerful ecological perspective. It acts on different states of consciousness, augmented by a variety of techniques, with the intention of making a voluntary and controlled transition to another state of conscious awareness (Money 2001). In this respect, all forms of ritual associated with intentional healing could be considered to promote an altered state of consciousness, whether this is by hand movements, the laying on of hands, meditation, meditative prayer, intercessionary prayer and liturgical prayer (Aldridge 2000), positive affirmation and so on.

Attitude and belief are directly linked to these processes, in that 'energy' is channelled in order to initiate a healing effect. Healing is almost always linked to a range of variables such as an individual's psychological profile and the way in which they interact with the environment and with other living beings. Ernst (2001) has suggested that there is no scientific evidence to support the existence of such 'energy', nor for any other concept underlying spiritual healing. However, Benor (1992, 2004) has undertaken some analysis of research into this field and argues that, whilst we may not understand the way in which this occurs, the effects of healing are 'beyond reasonable doubt'. A systematic review of 22 RCTs indicated that half of the studies found positive results (Abbot 2000, Astin et al 2000). More recently, Benor (2004) analysed 191 controlled

225

studies of healing. Of these, 124 demonstrated significant effects for healing; of 37 of the most rigorous studies reviewed, 23 showed an efficacy of more than 1:100 and the other 12 showed efficacy of greater than 3:100.

Diagnosis and treatment

Several treatments are usually required and a session may last up to 1 hour. Diagnosis is not really appropriate here but the healer may sweep his or her hands over the client's body, to detect, for example, temperature changes and thus focus on the area to be treated. A range of healing techniques may be employed. Distance or non-local healing may also occur, e.g. with prayer (Dossey 1993). A healer will discuss a problem with a patient and the patient may be healed lying down, standing or sitting. A mantra or prayer may be used and light direct hand touching or close proximity non-touch, where slow sweeping hand movements pass over the affected part or all of the body.

Box 5.1: **Healing approaches**

- *Spiritual healing:* laying on or close proximity of hands in which a special state of mind is required for healing to occur (Benor 1990, 2004)
- *Reiki:* an interactive approach where healing energy is transferred from healer to client with the aim of restoring health and harmony to the client's energy field (Rankin-Box 2001, Wirth et al 1993b)
- *Le Shan:* everyone has a natural ability for healing which can be accessed through the appropriate technique (Le Shan 1974)
- *Shamanism*: generally refers to specific tribes engaged in maintaining psychic and ecological equilibrium of their existence (Engebretson 1996, Graham 1991, Money 2001). May involve rhythmic swaying or chanting. Various forms described in Polynesia, China, South Pacific and the Americas

Box 5.2: **Common stages of healing techniques**

May occur locally, in close proximity to client or at a distance.

- *Centring*: initial preparation in which healer focuses upon care to be given
- *Assessment:* the healer may sweep hands over the client to detect, for example, temperature changes over the client's body, which may facilitate healing focus
- *Healing:* stroking or sweeping gestures across the body in an attempt to rebalance or redirect energy towards health

Box 5.3: **Indications for healing**

- Relief of postoperative pain after surgical removal of teeth (Wirth et al 1993a)
- Chronic pain
- Wound healing (Benor 2004, Wirth et al 1993b)
- Relaxation
- Anxiety
- Hypertension
- Emotional problems, including those associated with serious disease
- Spiritual welfare (Koenig et al 1998)
- Care of the elderly
- Caregivers of cancer patients

227

References and Further Reading

Abbot NC 2000 Healing as a therapy for human disease: a systematic review. Journal of Alternative and Complementary Medicine 6:159–169.

Aldridge D 2000 Spirituality, healing and medicine: return to the silence. Jessica Kingsley, London.

Astin J, Harkness E, Ernst E 2000 The efficacy of spiritual healing: a systematic review of randomised trials. Annals of Internal Medicine 132:903–910.

Benor DJ 1990 Survey of spiritual healing research. Complementary Medical Research 4:9–33.

Benor DJ 1992 Healing research: holistic energy medicine and spirituality. Vol I. Research into healing. Helix Editions, Oxford.

Benor DJ 2004 Consciousness, bioenergy and healing: self-healing and energy medicine for the 21st century. Healing Research Volume II. Wholistic Healing Publications, USA.

Dossey L 1993 Healing words: the power of prayer and the practice of medicine. Harper Collins, New York.

Engebretson J 1996 Urban healers: an experimental description of American healing touch groups. Qualitative Health Research 6(4):526–541.

Ernst E (ed) 2001 The desktop guide to complementary and alternative medicine: an evidence based approach. Mosby, Edinburgh.

Glik DC 1990 The redefinition of the situation in the social construction of spiritual healing experiences. Sociology of Health and Illness 12:151–168.

Graham H 1991 The return of the shaman: the emergence of the biophysical approach to health and healing. Complementary Medical Research 5(3):165–171.

Koenig HG, George LK, Hays JC, et al 1998 The relationship between religious activities and blood pressure in older adults. International Journal of Psychiatry in Medicine 28:189–213.

Le Shan L 1974 The medium, the mystic and the physicist: toward a general theory of the paranormal. Viking Press, New York.

Money M 2001 Shamanism. In: Rankin-Box D (ed) The nurse's handbook of complementary therapies. Baillière Tindall, Edinburgh.

National Center for Complementary and Alternative Medicine (NCCAM) 2002 Program announcements. Available online at: http://nccam.nih.gov/research/announcements/pa/index.html#active

Rankin-Box D 2001 Healing. In: Rankin-Box D (ed) The nurse's handbook of complementary therapies. Baillière Tindall, Edinburgh.

Struthers R, Eschiti VS, Patchell B 2004 Traditionasl indigenous healing: Part 1. Complementary Therapies in Nursing and Midwifery 10(3):141–149.

Wirth DP, Brenlan DR, Levine RJ, Rodriguez CM 1993a The effect of complementary healing therapy on postoperative pain after surgical removal of impacted third molar teeth. Complementary Therapies in Medicine 1:133–138.

Wirth DP, Richardson JT, Eidelman WC, O'Malley AC 1993b Full thickness dermal wounds treated with non-contact therapeutic touch: a replication and extension. Complementary Therapies in Medicine 1:127–132.

Hypnotherapy

Principles: hypnosis is the deliberate use of the trance state to effect change in both the conscious and unconscious states. The individual and *not* the therapist is considered to be in control of their trance state

Positive aspects: hypnotherapy is considered useful in anxiety, insomnia, stress-related disorders, phobias, pain and particularly in a range of addictions, including smoking and narcotics. Generally safe if practised ethically

Negative aspects: use of hypnosis as entertainment undermines the clinical efficacy of this approach and may result in misunderstanding concerning hynotherapy

General principles of hypnotherapy

Trance is commonly described as an altered state of consciousness or even day dreaming. This natural state may occur several times each day; however, the deliberate and conscious use of the trance state may be effective for a range of conditions. Hypnotic practices have existed in many cultures over the centuries, and hypnotism in the West was also initially referred to as 'mesmerism' (as popularized by Franz Mesmer).

During World War II, Simmel developed a technique called 'hypnoanalysis' for treating neurosis (Tamin 1988). James Braid is credited with enhancing the credibility of hypnosis to the medical community in the 1950s and the British and American Medical Associations now recognize hypnotherapy as a legitimate medical practice (Ernst 2001, Rankin-Box 2001). More recent developments in this field are described by Rankin-Box (2001), Erikson & Rossi (1980) and Spiegel & Spiegel (1978).

Hypnotherapy is commonly associated with the induction of a trance state during which behavioural modification may be suggested. Contrary to popular belief, the therapist does not take control of the client but acts only as a facilitator, helping a motivated individual towards a desired behavioural modification, e.g. smoking cessation. A positive desire by an individual to modify behaviour is central to success. 'Suggestion' refers to the presentation of an idea to a client and the extent to which a client accepts the idea ('suggestibility') is influenced by motivation and expectation. There is no definitive research to adequately explain this phenomenon. Whilst suggestion remains largely psychological or a placebo-like response, it is possible, using hypnotherapy, to anaesthetize parts of the body and influence the autonomic nervous system, which is not usually under voluntary control (Chakraverty et al 1992, Rankin-Box 2001, Whorewell et al 1992).

Diagnosis and treatment

Therapy typically lasts for 30–90 minutes per session. A general history is taken from the client identifying areas of concern. Commonly, clients are asked to focus on a 'point' and let their breathing become slow and relaxed. As their eyelids become heavy, they are asked to close them and guided visualization techniques may then be used. Trance is ended gradually, allowing the client to control the speed at which they emerge from their trance state. Reorientation may be facilitated by the therapist counting backwards, say from three to one. Descriptions of the trance state vary from 'an altered state of consciousness similar to a meditative state', 'deep relaxation' to 'a heightened state of awareness' (Rankin-Box 2001).

The precise way in which hypnosis occurs is still not fully understood. Whilst hypnotherapy is associated with deep relaxation, this rationale does not fully explain the ability of patients in trance to affect aspects of the autonomic nervous system such as bleeding, heart rate, gut peristalsis, skin temperature or irritable bowel syndrome (Harvey et al 1989) or to improve bronchial hyperresponsiveness in patients with moderate asthma (Ewer & Stewart 1986). Kirsch et al (1995) conducted a metaanalysis of 18 controlled trials and concluded that hypnotherapy enhanced the effects of cognitive (behavioural) psychotherapy for a range of conditions, including hypertension, anxiety, insomnia and pain. The use of hypnotherapy for smoking cessation has been questioned by Abbott et al (1998), who conducted a systematic review of nine RCTs of smoking cessation and concluded that hypnotherapy was no more effective than other treatments. However, studies into pain management with this therapy found a positive effect (Montgomery et al 2000, Rankin-Box 2001), including in paediatrics (Milling & Constantino 2000, Rankin-Box 2001).

Hypnotherapy has considerable potential for use within healthcare provision and is an increasingly accepted adjunct for a range of pain management conditions. The possible applications are wide ranging but whether it can be used effectively in the clinical setting depends largely upon the client's willingness to manage their own healthcare since the therapist is only a facilitator of the therapeutic process. Self-hypnosis may also be learnt by clients, enabling therapeutic self-sufficiency where appropriate and beneficial.

232

Box 5.4: **Stages of the hypnosis technique**

- *Induction:* linked to relaxation technique
- *Trigger:* may be used to induce deeper relaxation by suggestion
- *Deepening* (the ideomotor response): using, for example, finger movements or verbal responses
- *Therapy:* addressing client's concerns
- *Lightening:* reorientation to surroundings
- Ending: reorientation and end of trance state

Box 5.5: **Indications for hypnotherapy**

- Emesis for children receiving chemotherapy (Contach et al 1985)
- Control of peripheral skin temperature (Maslach et al 1972)
- Smoking cessation, including during pregnancy (Vaibo & Eide 1996)
- Irritable bowel syndrome (Harvey et al 1989, Whorewell et al 1992)
- Bronchial hyperresponsiveness in moderate asthma (Ewer & Stewart 1986)
- Pain management, including in paediatrics (Wadden & Anderton 1982)
- Stress management (Rankin-Box 2001, Tamin 1988)
- Postamputation phantom pain management (Rankin-Box 2001, Tamin 1988)
- Wound management (Rankin-Box 2001, Tamin 1988)
- Labour pain and relief of nausea (Rankin-Box 2001, Tamin 1988)
- Insomnia (Kirsch et al 1995)
- Anxiety, including that associated with dentistry
- Hypertension and obesity (Kirsch et al 1995)

Box 5.6: **Contraindications to hypnotherapy**

- Long-standing psychological problems
- Severe depression
- Borderline psychosis
- Has potential to retraumatize clients with posttraumatic disorder but this is rare if undertaken by a properly trained hypnotherapist

233

References and Further Reading

Abbott NC, Stead LF, White AR, Barnes J, Ernst E 1998 Hypnotherapy for smoking cessation (Cochrane Review). Cochrane Library. Update Software, Oxford.

Chakraverty K, Pharoah P, Scott D, Barker S 1992 Erythromyalgia: the role of hypnotherapy. Postgraduate Medical Journal 68:44–46.

Contach P, Hockenbury M, Herman S 1985 Self hypnosis as an anti-emetic therapy in children receiving chemotherapy. Oncology Nursing Forum 12:41–46.

Erikson M, Rossi E (eds) 1980 Innovative hypnotherapy – the collected works of Milton H Erikson on hypnosis. Vol. IV. Irvington, New York.

Ernst E (ed) 2001 The desktop guide to complementary and alternative medicine: an evidence based approach. Mosby, Edinburgh.

Ewer TC, Stewart DE 1986 Improvement of bronchial hyperresponsiveness in patients with moderate asthma after treatment with a hypnotic technique: a randomised controlled trial. British Medical Journal 293: 1129–1132.

Harvey RF, Gunary RM, Barry RE 1989 Individual and group hypnotherapy in treatment of refractory irritable bowel syndrome. Lancet i:424–425.

Kirsch I, Montgomery G, Sapirstein G 1995 Hypnosis as an adjunct to cognitive behavioural psychotherapy: a meta-analysis. Journal of Consulting and Clinical Psychology 63:214–220.

Maslach C, Marshall G, Zimbardo PG 1972 Hypnotic control of peripheral skin temperature: a case report. Psychophysiology 9:600–605.

Milling LS, Constantino CA 2000 Clinical hypnosis with children: first steps towards empirical support. International Journal of Clinical and Experimental Hypnotherapy 48:113–137.

Montgomery GH, Du Hamel KN, Redd WH 2000 A meta-analysis of hypnotically induced analgesia: how effective is hypnosis? International Journal of Clinical and Experimental Hypnotherapy 48:138–153.

Rankin-Box D 2001 Hypnosis. In: Rankin-Box D (ed) The nurse's handbook of complementary therapies. Baillière Tindall, Edinburgh.

Spiegel H, Spiegel D 1978 Trance and treatment: clinical uses of hypnosis. Basic Books, New York.

Tamin J 1988 Hypnosis. In: Rankin-Box D (ed) Complementary health therapies: a guide for nurses and the caring professions. Croom Helm, Beckenham, Kent.

Vaibo A, Eide T 1996 Smoking cessation in pregnancy: the effect of hypnosis in a randomised study. Addictive Behaviors 21:29–35.

Wadden TA, Anderton CGH 1982 The clinical use of hypnosis. Psychological Bulletin 91:215–243.

Whorewell PJ, Houghton L, Taylor E, Maxton D 1992 Physiological effects of emotion: assessment via hypnosis. Lancet 340:69–72.

Music therapy

Principles: the prescribed use of music in order to enhance, improve and maintain a therapeutic effect for physical and psychological well-being. Music can initiate emotional response and memory

Positive aspects: safe and pleasant; facilitates emotional well-being, social functioning, cognitive abilities and communication. Effective for children with learning disabilities, Alzheimer's disease and certain age-related problems

Negative aspects: selection of music for the client is critical and may be age related. Evidence suggests that some forms of music are aggressive, and violent lyrics may have negative effects upon an individual

General principles of music therapy

The concept of music as a positive healing influence for health and well-being can be traced back to Plato and Aristotle, who believed that music had the ability to promote health in mind and body. Followers of Pythagoras developed a science of music psychotherapy (Kayne 2002) and Homer claimed that music could help to avoid negative emotions (Standley 1998). Musical instruments have existed for thousands of years, during which magical powers were attributed to sound (Cowan 1992, McClellan 1991).

A distinction can be made between 'music therapy' and music *as* therapy. The former is practised by trained music therapists, whilst the latter may be used in a more informal manner to achieve significant improvements in health and well-being (Biley 2001). Autobiographical recall in patients with dementia can be considerably improved by music (Foster & Valentine 2001) and it is believed that music creates a level of coherence between the electrical activities of different areas of the brain. Music was also used in the form of incantations, songs, rhythms and sounds, to ward off evil spirits, absolve sins and placate the gods (Alvin 1966).

In ancient Egypt, music was regarded as the 'physic of the soul' (Biley 2001). Early experiments into the therapeutic uses of music were published in the 18th century by Dogiel, who suggested that music induced physiological responses enhancing circulation of the blood. In 1896, Patrici demonstrated that blood circulation to the brain could be slowed and reduced by the effects of music. During the first and second world wars, music was recognized as a therapeutic tool and musicians were hired by hospitals. In 1944 the first music therapy degree was established in Michigan State University. For many contemporary societies and social groups, music continues to be associated with such qualities and forms a central aspect of social structure and social cohesion.

Barnason et al (1995) described research which indicated consistent improvements in the psychological state of participants upon exposure to music. In particular, listening to Mozart's Sonata for Two Pianos (K448) significantly enhanced the ability of subjects to perform spatial awareness tests (Rauscher et al 1995). There are indicators that positive physiological responses to music exist, which are measurable through pulse rate, blood pressure, electroencephalograph and galvanic skin response (GSR) (Thaut 1990, Watkins 1997). A controlled study of 40 babies, to whom lullabies were sung and who were massaged once a week until discharge, demonstrated shorter hospital stays by an average of 11 days for female and 1.5 days for male infants, indicating sex differences as well as the benefits of listening to music (Standley 1998).

Box 5.7: **Indications for music therapy**

- Improvements in spatial awareness (certain types of music; Rauscher et al 1995)
- As displacement activity to reduce feelings of anxiety and uncertainty
- Reduction of neonatal hospital stay
- Alternative channel of communication for, e.g., autistic children and those with attention deficit hyperactivity disorder (ADHD; Bunt 1999)
- Enhanced survival in patients with serious disease (Marwick 2000)
- Enhanced recall in patients with dementia
- Reduction of pain and anxiety in a hospital setting (Koch et al 1998, Winter et al 1994)

Box 5.8: **Precautions**

- Choice of music is critical
- Music preferences can be influenced by culture, age and medical condition (e.g. pain relief, relaxation, coordination)
- Some religious faiths, or divisions of these, may not approve (e.g. music has occasionally been described as 'un-Islamic')
- Increased memory recall may initiate negative as well as positive memories (McCraty et al 1998)

238

Diagnosis and treatment

Music therapy consists of listening to music to stimulate a therapeutic physiological or psychological response. The therapeutic benefits of listening to music relate strongly to the type of music being played, the quality of the music and the environment in which it is heard. In music therapy, licences from, for example, the Performing Arts Society may be required.

References and Further Reading

Alvin J 1996 Music therapy. J Baker, London.

Barnason S, Zimmerman L, Nieveen J 1995 The effects of music intervention on anxiety in the patient after coronary artery bypass grafting. Heart and Lung 24(2):124–132.

Biley F 2001 Music as therapy. In: Rankin-Box D (ed) The nurse's handbook of complementary therapies. Baillière Tindall, Edinburgh.

Bunt L 1999 Music therapy: an art beyond words. Routledge, London.

Cowan JG 1992 The Aboriginal tradition. Element, Shaftesbury, Dorset.

Foster NA, Valentine ER 2001 The effect of auditory stimulation on autobiographical recall in dementia. Experimental Aging Research 27:215–223.

Kayne SB 2002 Complementary therapies for pharmacists. Pharmaceutical Press, London.

Koch ME, Kain ZN, Ayoub C, Rosenbaum SH 1998 The sedative and analgesic sparing effect of music. Anesthesiology 89:300–306.

Marwick C 2000 Music therapists chime in with data on medical results. Journal of the American Medical Association 283:731–733.

McClellan R 1991 The healing forces of music: history, theory and practice. Element, Massachusetts.

McCraty R, Barrios-Chopin B, Atkinson M, Tomasino D 1998 The effects of different types of music on mood, tension and mental clarity. Alternative Therapies in Health and Medicine 4(1):75–84.

Rauscher FH, Shaw GL, Ky KN 1995 Listening to Mozart enhances spatial-temporal reasoning: towards a neurophysiological basis. Neurosci Lett 185:44–47.

Standley JM 1998 The effect of music and multimodal stimulation on responses of premature infants in neonatal intensive care. Paediatric Nurse 24:532–538.

Thaut MH 1990 Physiological and motor responses to music stimuli. In: Unekefer RF (ed) Music therapy in the treatment of adults with mental disorders. Schirmer Books, New York.

Watkins GR 1997 Music therapy: proposed physiological mechanisms and clinical implications. Clinical Nurse Specialist 11(2):43–50.

Winter MJ, Paskin S, Baker T 1994 Music reduces stress and anxiety of patients in the surgical holding area. Journal of Post Anaesthesia Nursing 9:340–343.

Website information

The following websites have been selected in order to provide readers with additional information and further contact details for particular therapies. The authors cannot vouch for the accuracy of the information contained within the websites.

It is believed that website addresses are generally more consistent than postal addresses and provide faster information access routes. This list is not exhaustive and readers are advised to monitor developments and information emerging in the field of CAM.

COMPLEMENTARY MEDICINE (GENERAL)

British Holistic Medical Association
www.bhma.org

Research Council for Complementary Medicine
www.rccm.org.uk

Institute of Complementary Medicine
www.i-c-m.org.uk

Prince of Wales's Foundation for Integrated Health (POWFIH)
www.fihealth.org.uk

National Center for Complementary and Alternative Medicine: Complementary and Alternative Medicine in the US
www.http:/nccam.nih.gov

Complementary Medicine Addresses and Information
www.nassdb.org.uk/f2/Complementary_Medicine_Links_3.htm

Alternative and Complementary Medicine Directory
www.outsiders.org.uk/directory/04_alternative.htm

ACUPUNCTURE

British Acupuncture Council
www.acupuncture.org.uk

American Academy of Medical Acupuncture
www.medicalacupuncture.org

British Medical Acupuncture Society
www.medical-acupuncture.co.uk

International Veterinary Acupuncture Association
www.ivas.org/main.cfm

AROMATHERAPY

Aromatherapy Organisations Council (AOC)
www.aocuk.net

Aromatherapy Consortium
www.aromatherapy-regulation.org.uk

International Federation of Aromatherapists (IFA)
www.ifaroma.org

AUTOGENIC THERAPY

British Autogenic Society
www.autogenic-therapy.co.uk

Autogenic Society
www.autogenic-therapy.org.uk

BACH FLOWER REMEDIES

www.bachcentre.com

BIOFEEDBACK

Biofeedback Research Bibliography
www.cliving.org/biblobiof.htm

Biofeedback Foundation of Europe
www.bfe.org

HERBAL MEDICINE

British Herbal Medicine Association (BHMA)
www.exeter.ac.uk/phytonet/bhma.html

National Institute of Medical Herbalists
www.nimh.org.uk

Medline plus: a service of the US National Library of Medicine and National Institutes of Health
www.nlm.gov/medlineplus/herbalmedicine.html

Weleda Ltd
www.weleda.co.uk

Potter's Herbal Medicines
www.pottersherbals.co.uk/

HOMEOPATHY

243

www.internathealthlibrary.com/therapies/homeopathy-research.html

Faculty of Homeopathy London
www.trusthomeopathy.org/faculty

Faculty of Homeopathy Academic Department, Glasgow Homeopathic Hospital
www.trusthomeopathy.org/faculty *or* www.adhom.com

Society of Homeopaths
www.homeopathy-soh.com

Demystifying Homeopathy
www.homeopathicmedicalclinic.com/homeopathy/book_english/Safety.htm

Boiron
www.boiron.com/index_en.asp

British Institute of Homeopathy Ltd
www.britinsthom.com

Society of Homeopaths
www.homeopathy-soh.org

Homeopathic Medical Association
www.the-hma.org

Ainsworths
www.ainsworths.com/arf/arf.aspx

Helios
www.helios.co.uk

Nelsons Homeopathy and Bach Flower Remedies
www.nelsonbach.com/en.html

Weleda Ltd
www.weleda.co.uk

ABC Homeopathy (a good all-round website for advice)
www.abchomeopathy.com

HUMOUR AND LAUGHTER

General information
www.ncbi.nlm.nih.gov/entrez/query.fcgi?cmd=Retrieve
& db=PubMed&list_uids=9456713&dopt=Abstract

American Association for Therapeutic Humor
www.aath.org

Humor therapy
www.holistic-online.com/Humor_therapy_benefits.htm

HYPNOSIS

British Association of Hypnotists (BAH)
www.belmont-centre.co.uk

British Society of Medical and Dental Hypnosis (BSMDH)
www.bsmdh.org

American Society of Clinical Hypnosis
www.asch.net

National Register of Hypnotherapists and Psychotherapists
www.patient.co.uk/showdoc/26739023

MASSAGE

American Massage Therapy Association
www.amtamassage.org

Massage Therapy
www.massagetherapy.co.uk/default.asp?article=associations_prof

245

MUSIC THERAPY

General information
www.psychiatrictimes.com/p990246.html

American Society for Music Therapy
www.musictherapy.org/about.html

British Society for Music Therapy
www.bsmt.org

American Music Therapy Association
www.musictherapy.org

NATUROPATHY

General Council and Register of Naturopaths
www.naturopathy.org.uk

British College of Naturopathy and Osteopathy
www.bcno.ac.uk *or*
www.merlinhelpsstudents.com/universities/BritishColle
geOfNaturopathyAndOsteopathy.asp

British Naturopathic Association
www.naturopaths.org.uk/default.asp

OSTEOPATHY

General Osteopathic Council (GOC)
www.osteopathy.co.uk

British College of Osteopathy
www.bcom.ac.uk/of

REFLEXOLOGY

General information
www.wolist.com/wo/health/alternative/reflexology

Association of Reflexologists (AoR)
www.reflexology.org

International Council of Reflexologists
www.icr-reflexology.org

RELAXATION AND VISUALIZATION

General information
www.monte.wednet.edu/sports/baseball/relaxation_&_
visualization.htm

Multiple Sclerosis Society
www.nationalmssociety.org/spotlight-relax.asp

Guided imagery
www.guidedimageryinc.com/stress.html

SHIATSU

**Shiatsu and Lifestyle Experience: Shiatsu Society
resources**
www.bssf-shiatsu-do.co.uk/directory/shiatsu-society.
html

Shiatsu Society
www.shiatsu.org

Innerself
www.innerself.com/Health/discovering_shiatsu.htm

Medline
http://holisticonline.com/Shiatsu/hol_shiatsu_home.htm

SPIRITUAL HEALING

National Federation of Spiritual Healers (NFSH)
www.nfsh.org.uk

Sacred Space Foundation
www.sacredsites.com

Holistic healing research
www.holistichealingresearch.com

General research
www.siib.org.Downloads/Sciencespiritual.pdf

THERAPEUTIC TOUCH

Sacred Space Foundation
www.therapeutic-touch.org
www.energy-healing.7gen.com

Medline
http://altmed.creighton.edu/touch/favorite.htm

Glossary

Acupuncture – Latin *acus* (needle) and *punctara* (puncture). An ancient form of healthcare practice and medicine which aims to treat illness and maintain health through the stimulation of the body's self-healing powers. May involve use of fine needles to stimulate or unblock energy (Qi) flow around the body, herbs, moxibustion, diet, exercise; with the intention to restore harmony, energy balance and maintain health in the body.

Alexander Technique – the use of conscious posture and breathing pattern modification to enhance health and well-being. AT is based upon the premise that poor body posture can contribute towards ill health and chronic pain.

Anthroposophical medicine – perception of health and disease wherein the soul and spirit are said to affect health. It is believed that there are four manifestations of the body and three systems by which they can function. Approach developed by Rudolf Steiner who claimed health is maintained when the three systems are in harmony.

Aromatherapy – the therapeutic use of fragrances derived from plants and flowers to produce essential oils. These may be inhaled, ingested (rarely) or combined with a carrier oil for application through skin massage.

Art therapy – the therapeutic use of art, drawing, painting or sculpting to facilitate emotional expression and mood enhancement. Sculpture and modelling may be used in certain psychiatric settings as a form or expressionism or, for example, to develop concentration.

Autogenic training – a psychophysiological therapy combining relaxation and self-hypnosis in order to train an individual to enter a relaxed receptive state through which mental and physical homeostasis (rebalancing) may occur.

Ayurveda – an indigenous form of Indian medicine based on an ancient system of balance and harmony epitomized by the Tridosha; uses traditional formulae and mixtures of herbs and minerals, has a great emphasis on cleansing the system. The term is derived from *ayur*, meaning life or longevity, and *veda*, meaning knowledge. Ayurvedic medicine can involve a range of procedures including nutrition, exercise, yoga and herbal medicines. A related, more practical form of folk medicine is *unani-tibb* or *unani*. *Related techniques include: herbalism, unani-tibb.*

Bach Flower Remedies – the use of distilled essences of wild flowers taken diluted in water or spirit or as a lotion. The therapy is based on the premise that disease is directly related to temperament; thus remedies treat anxiety, insomnia or disharmony.

Biodynamic massage – see Massage.

Biofeedback – a method of operant conditioning whereby an individual learns to control otherwise involuntary body functions such as heart rate, blood pressure, headaches, insomnia.

Bowen Technique – gentle soft tissue manipulation. May be used for stress relief and anxiety. *Related techniques include: massage, shiatsu.*

Centring – an initial stage of practitioner preparation in which they become relaxed and focused on the care about to be given. This activity is described by a number of therapies such as massage, reiki and shiatsu.

Chelation therapy – a method used in naturopathy for removing toxins, metabolic wastes and minerals from the bloodstream using intravenous ethylene diamine tetraacetic acid (EDTA).

Chiropractic – specializes in the diagnosis and treatment of mechanical disorders of joints and their effects on the nervous system. Chiropractic employs a technique of spinal manipulation based upon the theory that problems associated with vertebral alignment may result in neural, muscular or sensory disorders. Realignment of the spine aims to restore normal movement through manipulation.

Cognitive therapy – a form of psychotherapy using imagery, self-instruction and related techniques to alter distorted attitudes and perception.

Colour therapy – the use of colour in lighting, paints or materials to help ameliorate physical and psychological problems.

Complementary medicine – a generic term referring to a range of therapeutic modalities currently perceived as adjuncts to orthodox medicine. More recently, the terms 'integrated medicine' and 'integrated health' have been promoted as increasing numbers of therapies demonstrate scientific efficacy and become integrated within mainstream medicine. *Related techniques include: alternative, integrated medicine, integrated health.*

Counselling skills – a repertoire of verbal and non-verbal communication skills employed to promote psychological well-being in order to help clients to identify and clarify life experiences or problems and to support them.

251

Crystal therapy – the belief that minerals and rocks possess therapeutic forms of energy that can be harnessed to promote well-being. *Related techniques include: stone therapy, colour therapy.*

Doshas –the three basic forces or humours, *Vata, Pitta and Kapha,* in Ayurvedic medicine.

Electrodermal response (EDR) – a means of measuring general levels of autonomic arousal commonly used in biofeedback.

Essential oil – undiluted oil extracted from various parts of plants and flowers, commonly diluted in a carrier oil before use.

Functional food – food that has been modified, processed or otherwise had incorporated into it a natural component to give it a specific medical or health benefit.

Geopathic stress – a theory that energies emanate from the earth, manifesting through stress or ley lines, which may affect general health and well-being.

Hara diagnosis – a form of diagnosis used in shiatsu and a number of Eastern cultures, involving gentle palpation of the abdominal region. In shiatsu, the *hara* is also referred to as the *tandien,* the centre of balance and gravity.

Healing – therapeutic form of energy exchange based upon a cause-and-effect relationship between a healer's conscious intention (conscious intentionality) to heal and subsequent improvement in client symptoms and physical and psychological well-being. The term may also be used generically to describe specific 'healing' practices. *Related techniques include: therapeutic touch, non-contact touch, spiritual healing, laying on of hands, meditation, reiki.*

Herbal medicine – the use of decoctions of herb and plant material by trained practitioners to facilitate healing and health. Subcategories include botanical medicine, Chinese herbalism, Ayurveda, kampo, phytotherapy and rational phytotherapy.

Holism – relating to a theory of wholeness. Holistic medicine and holism consider that individuals function as a whole rather than as a combination of separate systems. Thus mind, body and spirit are interrelated.

Homeopathy – a system of medicine based upon the Law of Similars (let like be treated with like). Effectivity is obtained through a process of dilution during which extracts from natural sources such as plants and minerals are diluted many times in a water and alcohol base. At each dilution the mixture is succussed (vigorously shaken). Homeopaths believe that succussion enhances the potency of dilution. Homeopathy may be given in liquid form or by tablets. *Related techniques include: bioemic medicine, isopathy, tautopathy.*

Humour and laughter therapy – a psychological intervention based upon humour or an amusing intervention designed to be of benefit to the patient. Can be effective in increasing cortisol levels and pain reduction. *Related techniques include: displacement therapy, visualization, hypnosis.*

Hypnosis – the deliberate use of the trance state to effect change in the conscious (e.g. breathing) and/or autonomic nervous system (gut peristalsis, blood pressure). A principle of hypnosis is that the individual is in control of their trance state and not the hypnotist. Thus hypnosis is fundamentally self-hypnosis with the therapist acting as a facilitator. *Related techniques include: visualization, biofeedback, meditation.*

Iridology – a diagnostic tool based on the assumption that examination of the iris can indicate the general status of internal organs.

Kinesiology – a therapy based on traditional acupuncture theory to determine structural or chemical dysfunction. It is believed that such dysfunction can be diagnosed via secondary muscle

253

imbalance. Treatment occurs through manipulation of the cranium and body joints.

Massage – the conscious, deliberate and often formalized soft tissue manipulation of the body using pressure, light kneading or traction to promote relaxation and well-being. *Related techniques include: Swedish massage, biomassage, shiatsu, aromatherapy, reflexology, Indian head massage, reiki.*

Meridians – conceptual channels through which Qi (yin/yang) energy is said to flow around the body. Imbalance in energy flow is referred to as a blockage (build-up or stagnation of energy (yang) or deficiency of energy (yin)). Meridian channels are accessed through points on the body surface (*tsubos*) and treated in acupuncture with fine needles and in shiatsu via direct fingertip pressure (see Acupuncture and Shiatsu).

Moxibustion (jiu) – related to acupuncture and acupressure. Involves use of heat in the form of smouldering leaves of, for example, mugwort (*Artemisia vulgaris*) rolled into various shapes or cones. These may be attached to the distal end of the needle whilst it is in position, so transmitting heat along the needle to the acupuncture point. Alternatively a cone may be applied directly over a point and lit; this is said to stimulate energy.

Music therapy – the use of music in order to enhance, improve and maintain a therapeutic effect for physical and psychological well-being.

Naturopathy – a multidisciplinary approach to healthcare founded on a belief in the power of the body to heal itself.

Neurolinguistic programming – the use of learnt behavioural strategies and changes to thought patterns to assist problem solving. Effective for anxiety, stress and personal development. *Related techniques include: hypnosis, meditation, relaxation, imagery.*

Nutraceuticals – products produced from food, but presented in a form not usually associated with food (e.g. tablets, capsules) used as medicines to prevent or treat diseases. *Related techniques include: diet, naturopathy.*

Nutritional therapy – based on the assumption that the state of one's health is directly contingent upon what is eaten. Nutritional therapy focuses upon the effects certain foods have on health and illness. *Related techniques include: diet, nutraceuticals.*

Osteopathy – a system of manual medicine concerned with mechanical, functional and postural treatment. Osteopathy involves manipulation of joints and spinal vertebrae aimed at resolving mechanical problems of the body. Osteopaths believe that the central role of the physician is to facilitate self-healing.

Placebo effect – a therapeutic effect that can occur after the administration of a placebo (an inert substance or intervention) that initiates a physiological or psychological response.

Placebo response – self-healing response.

Polarity therapy – an energy-based system involving bodywork, diet, exercise and lifestyle counselling aimed at maintaining and balancing energy flows through the body. Polarity therapy is based on the premise that all energy within the human body is grounded in electromagnetic forces, with disease resulting from poorly dissipated energy.

Prakruti – the human constitution in Ayurveda, determined by the state of the parental Tridosha at conception. Expressed as Vata, Pitta or Kapha types although most people are not completely one type

255

but can be described as Vata-Pitta or Pitta-Kapha, for example.

Prana – the essential life force in Ayurveda.

Process of counselling – occurs within a non-directive therapeutic relationship. Clients are enabled to self-actualize and develop their own abilities to resolve or accept situations.

Qi (pronounced 'chi') – the essential life force in Traditional Chinese Medicine.

Qi-Gong – a branch of the Chinese medical system integrating exercise, self-massage, structured movements and meditation to enhance Qi energy. *Related techniques include: Tai Chi, shiatsu, reiki.*

Reflexology – a treatment which applies varying degrees of pressure, commonly to the hands and feet, to promote health and well-being based upon the premise that the internal organs of the body are mapped out on the surface of these organs. Treatment occurs through gentle pressure to specific areas of the hands or feet, which effect a change elsewhere in the body through 'reflexes or zones' that run along the body. *Related techniques include: massage, shiatsu, reiki.*

Reiki – Japanese healing discipline derived from the Usui natural healing system (also known as *Usui shiki ryoko*) involving the laying on of hands. Reiki may be translated as 'healing'; *Rei* means 'universal'; *ki* (Qi) means 'life force energy'.

Relaxation – a state of altered consciousness characterized by the release of muscular tension, anxiety and stress. Can also elicit a relaxation response of the autonomic nervous system. Process involves progressive muscular relaxation. Relaxation exercises are frequently incorporated into healthcare practice and antenatal care. *Related techniques include: visual guided imagery, autogenic training, hypnosis, biofeedback, yoga, meditation.*

Shiatsu – literally means 'finger pressure'. A physical therapy grounded in Japanese culture based upon the same premise as acupuncture but rather than using fine needles to stimulate and harmonize Qi energy flow around the body, shiatsu practitioners direct pressure to key points (*tsubos*) to promote health and well-being. *Related techniques include: acupuncture, moxibustion, reiki, massage.*

Succussion – a process employed in homeopathy whereby natural diluted substances are vigorously shaken. Homeopaths believe that this process augments the healing potency of dilutions.

Swedish massage – a system combining exercise and massage to treat joint and muscular problems based upon the premise that vigorous massage could promote health and healing by enhancing circulation of blood and lymph.

Tai Chi – a process of systematic slow martial art movements and physical postures to promote flexibility, focus and harmony.

Therapeutic touch (TT) – described as an energy field interaction between two or more people with the intention to rebalance or repattern the energy field in order to facilitate relaxation and self-healing. See also Healing. *Related techniques include: healing, spiritual healing, non-touch healing, visualization.*

Traditional Chinese Medicine – based upon a sophisticated and ancient system of balance and harmony epitomized by yin and yang; uses traditional formulae and mixtures of herbs, plus other non-drug treatment such as acupuncture.

Trance – an altered state of consciousness.

257

Tridosha – a collective term for the three doshas, the basic forces or humours Vata, Pitta and Kapha, in Ayurveda.

Visualization – use of imagination and psychological imagery to positively influence health. For example, anxiety reduction, insomnia, panic attacks, management of pain.

Yin/yang – philosophical concept underpinning therapies such as acupuncture and shiatsu. Yin and yang energy is described as a dynamic symbiotic relationship between active and passive energy forces said to be present in the universe and the human body. Yang energy is characterized by symptoms related to heat, movement, activity and excess; Yin energy relates generally to symptoms of cold, sluggishness, inactivity and deficiency. A balance of each kind of energy is necessary for health. Rather like the scales of justice, an excess of yin energy results in depletion of yang energy and vice versa. The aim is to maintain harmonious balance between the two forces. *Related techniques include: acupuncture, shiatsu, reiki.*

Yoga – the practice of gentle structured breathing, meditation and stretching exercises to promote flexibility and relaxation. Yoga is derived from the Sanskrit word *yuj* meaning 'to yoke'. The purpose is to join the mind to the body through harmonious breathing, meditation and physical exercise. The main yoga practices used in the West are breath control (*pranayama*), meditation and poses (*asanas*). *Related techniques include: Tai Chi, meditation.*

Zones – a reflexology term describing how the body's innate energy (Qi) is said to flow through reflexes that terminate in the hands or feet.

Qualification abbreviations

Please note that this list is not exhaustive; new qualifications are being recognized all the time.

ABAH	Associate of the British Hypnotherapy Association
ABATH	Associate of the British Association of Therapeutical Hypnotists
ABMAc	Associate of the British Medical Acupuncture Society
ABT	Association of Bodymind Therapists
AIRMT	Associate of the International Register of Manipulative Therapists
AMA	Anthroposophical Medical Association
AMP	Association of Massage Practitioners
ANLP	Association for NLP
APMT(GB)	Association of Professional Music Therapists in Great Britain
ATA	Association of Tisserand Aromatherapists
ATAcS	Associate of the Traditional Acupuncture Society
BAAR	British Acupuncture Association and Register
BCA	British Chiropractic Association
BHMA	British Holistic Medical Association
BPsS	British Society of Psychotherapists
BRCP	British Register of Complementary Practitioners
CAc	Certificate of Acupuncture (China)
CCAc	Certificate in Chinese Acupressure
CertHS	Certificate in Herbal Studies

CHP	Certificate in Hypnotherapy and Psychotherapy (National College of Hypnosis and Psychotherapy)
CHyp	Certified Hypnotherapist (Member of the British Council of Hypnotist Examiners)
CHyp	Council of Hypnotherapies
CMH	Certified Master Hypnotist (Member of the British Council of Hypnotist Examiners)
DAc	Diploma in Acupuncture (College of Traditional Chinese Acupuncture)
DC	Diploma in Chiropractic
DHM	Diploma in Holistic Medicine
DHom	Diploma in Homeopathy
DHP	Diploma in Hypnotherapy and Psychotherapy
DipC	Diploma in Counselling
DipHyp	Diploma in Hypnotherapy
DipPhyt	Diploma in Phytotherapy (herbal medicine)
DipTHP	Diploma in Therapeutic Hypnosis and Psychotherapy
DO	Diploma in Osteopathy
DrAc	Doctor of Acupuncture (British College of Acupuncture)
DSH	Diploma from the School of Homeopathy
DTM	Diploma in Therapeutic Massage
FbcA	Fellow of the British Acupuncture Association
FFHom	Fellow of the Faculty of Homeopathy
FLCO	Fellow of the London College of Osteopaths
FNIMH	Fellow of the National Institute of Medical Herbalists
FRH	Fellow of the Register of Herbalists
IRNHP	Independent Register of Natural Health Practitioners
ISPA	International Society of Practising Aromatherapists
LCCH	London College of Classical Homeopathy

LCH	Licentiate of the College of Homeopathy
LCHom	Licentiate of the College of Homeopaths
LCSP(Chir)	Licentiate of the Chartered Society of Physiotherapists (Chiropody)
LCSP(Phys)	Licentiate of the Chartered Society of Physiotherapists (Remedial Massage and Manipulative Therapy)
LicAc	Licentiate in Acupuncture
LicAc(AWA)	Licentiate of the Academy of Western Acupuncture
LNCP	Licentiate of National Council of Psychotherapists
MAA	Member of the Auricular Therapy Association
MAc	Master of Acupuncture
MACH	Member of the Association of Classical Hypnotherapists
MAR	Member of the Association of Reflexologists
MAWAc	Member of the Association of Western Acupuncture
MBAcA	Member of the British Acupuncture Association
MBEOA	Member of the British European Osteopathic Association
MBNOA	Member of the British Naturopathic and Osteopathic Association
MBRA	Member of the British Reflexology Association
MBRI	Member of the British Register of Iridologists
MBSAM	Member of the British School of Acupressure
MBSH	Member of the British Society of Hypnotherapists
MBSR	Member of the British School of Reflexology

MC	McTimoney Chiropractor
MCH	Member of the College of Homeopathy
MCO	Member of the College of Osteopaths
MCOA	Member of the College of Healing
MCROA	Member of the Cranial Osteopathic Association
MFG	Member of the Feldenkrais Guild
MFHom	Member of the Faculty of Homeopathy
MGNM	Member of the Guild of Natural Medicine Practitioners
MGO	Member of the Guild of Osteopathy
MGPMP	Member of the Guild of Professional Massage Practitioners
MH	Master Herbalist
MHPA	Member of the Health Practitioners Association
MIACT	Member of the International Association of Colour Therapists
MIAH	Member of the Institute of Analytical Hypnotherapists
MIAO	Member of the Institute of Applied Osteopathy
MICH	Member of the Institute of Curative Hypnotherapists
MIFA	Member of the International Federation of Aromatherapists
MIGN(Med)	Member of the International Guild of Natural Medicine Practitioners
MIIR	Member of the International Institute of Reflexology
MinstAT	Member of the Institute of Allergy Therapists
MIPC	Member of the Institute of Pure Chiropractic
MIPM	Member of the Institute of Psionic Medicine (Psionic Medical Society)
MIPTI	Member of the Independent Professional Therapists International

MIRMT	Member of the Independent Register of Manipulative Therapists
MIROM	Member of the International Register of Oriental Medicine
MISMA	Member of the International Stress Management Association
MISPH	Member of the International Society for Professional Hypnosis
MISPT	Member of the International Society of Polarity Therapists
MLCO	Member of the London College of Osteopathic Medicine
MMSM	Member of the Midlands School of Massage
MNAHP	Member of the National Association of Hypnotists and Psychotherapists
MNCPHR	Member of the National Council of Psychotherapists and Hypnotherapy Register
MNIMH	Member of the National Institute of Medical Herbalists
MNTOS	Member of the Natural Therapeutic and Osteopathic Society
MPNLP	Master Practitioner of NLP
MRadA	Member of the Radionics Association
MRCHM	Member of the Register of Chinese Herbal Medicine
MRCMT	Member of the Register of Chinese Massage Therapy
MRCN	Member of the Register of Clinical Nutritionists
MRH	Member of the Register of Herbalists
MRN	Member of the General Council and Register of Naturopaths
MRO	Member of the Register of Osteopaths
MRSS	Member of the Register of the Shiatsu Society
MRTCM	Member of the Register of Traditional Chinese Medicine

MSAA	Member of the Society of Auricular Acupuncturists
MSAPP	Member of the Society of Advanced Psychotherapists and Parapsychologists
MSBTh	Member of the Society of Health and Beauty Therapists
MSHP	Member of the Society of Holistic Practitioners
MO	Member of the Society of Osteopaths (European School of Osteopathy)
MSS	Member of the Shiatsu Society
MSTAT	Member of the Society of Teachers of the Alexander Technique
MTAcS	Member of the Traditional Acupuncture Society
MWFH	Member of the World Federation of Hypnotherapists
ND	Diploma in Naturopathy
NFSH	National Federation of Spiritual Healers
NRHP	National Register of Hypnotherapists and Psychotherapists
RIr	Registered Iridologist
RMANM	Registered Member of the Association of Natural Medicines
RMAPC	Registered Member of the Association of Psychic Counsellors
RNTOS	Register of the Natural Therapeutic and Osteopathic Society
RPT	Registered Polarity Therapist
RSHom	Register of the Society of Homoeopaths
RTCM	Register of Traditional Chinese Medicine
SAPP	Society of Advanced Psychotherapy Practitioners
SMD	Swedish Massage Diploma
TDHA	Tisserand Diploma in Holistic Aromatherapy

For further information on new qualifications please contact:

Institute for Complementary Medicine (ICM), PO Box 194, London SE16 7QZ

Tel: 020 7237 5165. Fax: 020 7237 5175. E-mail: icm@icmedicine.co.uk

Website: www.icmedicine.com

Normal blood values

Test	Reference range (conventional units)
Acidity (pH)	7.35–7.45
Alcohol	0 mg/dL (more than 0.1 mg/dL normally indicates intoxication) (ethanol)
Ammonia	15–50 µg of nitrogen/dL
Amylase	53–123 units/L
Ascorbic acid	0.4–1.5 mg/dL
Bicarbonate	18–23 mEq/L (carbon dioxide content)
Bilirubin	Direct: up to 0.4 mg/dL Total: up to 1.0 mg/dL
Blood volume	8.5–9.1% of total body weight
Calcium	8.5–10.5 mg/dL (normally slightly higher in children)
Carbon dioxide pressure	35–45 mmHg
Carbon monoxide	Less than 5% of total haemoglobin
CD4 cell count	500–1500 cells/µL
Caeruloplasmin	15–60 mg/dL
Chloride	98–106 mEq/L
Complete blood cell count (CBC)	Tests include: haemoglobin, haematocrit, mean corpuscular haemoglobin, mean corpuscular haemoglobin concentration, mean corpuscular volume, platelet count, white blood cell count
Copper	Total: 70–150 µg/dL
Creatine kinase (CK or CPK)	Male: 38–174 units/L Female: 96–140 units/L
Creatine kinase isoenzymes	5% MB or less
Creatinine	0.6–1.2 mg/dL
Electrolytes	Test includes: calcium, chloride, magnesium, potassium, sodium

Test	Reference range (conventional units)
Erythrocyte sedimentation rate (ESR or sed-rate)	Male: 1–13 mm/h Female: 1–20 mm/h
Glucose	Tested after fasting: 70–110 mg/dL
Haematocrit	Male: 45–62% Female: 37–48%
Haemoglobin	Male: 13–18 g/dL Female: 12–16 g/dL
Iron	60–160 µg/dL (normally higher in males)
Iron-binding capacity	250–460 µg/dL
Lactate (lactic acid)	Venous: 4.5–19.8 mg/dL Arterial: 4.5–14.4 mg/dL
Lactic dehydrogenase	50–150 units/L
Lead	40 µg/dL or less (normally much lower in children)
Lipase	10–150 units/L
Zinc B-Zn	70–102 µmol/L

Lipids:
  Cholesterol
 	
  Triglycerides
	Less than 225 mg/dL (for age 40–49 years; increases with age)
	
	10–29 years 53–104 mg/dL
	30–39 years 55–115 mg/dL
	40–49 years 66–139 mg/dL
	50–59 years 75–163 mg/dL
	60–69 years 78–158 mg/dL
	>70 years 83–141 mg/dL

Liver function tests	Tests include bilirubin (total), phosphatase (alkaline), protein (total and albumin), transaminases (alanine and aspartate), prothrombin (PTT)
Magnesium	1.5–2.0 mEq/L
Mean corpuscular haemoglobin (MCH)	27–32 pg/cell
Mean corpuscular haemoglobin concentration (MCHC)	32–36% haemoglobin/cell
Mean corpuscular volume (MCV)	76–100 cu µm

Osmolality	280–296 mOsm/kg water
Oxygen pressure	83–100 mmHg
Oxygen saturation (arterial)	96–100%
Phosphatase, prostatic	0–3 units/dL (Bodansky units) (acid)
Phosphatase	50–160 units/L (normally higher in infants and adolescents) (alkaline)
Phosphorus	3.0–4.5 mg/dL (inorganic)
Platelet count	150,000–350,000/mL
Potassium	3.5–5.0 mEq/L
Prostate-specific antigen (PSA)	0–4 ng/mL (likely higher with age)

Proteins:
   Total
   Albumin
   Globulin
	
	 6.0–8.4 g/dL
	 3.5–5.0 g/dL
	 2.3–3.5 gm/dL

Prothrombin (PTT)	25–41 sec
Pyruvic acid	0.3–0.9 mg/dL
Red blood cell count (RBC)	4.2–6.9 million/μL/cu mm
Sodium	135–145 mEq/L
Thyroid-stimulating hormone (TSH)	0.5–6.0 μ units/mL

Transaminases:
   Alanine (ALT)
   Aspartate (AST)
	
	 1–21 units/L
	 7–27 units/L

Urea nitrogen (BUN) BUN/creatinine ratio	7–18 mg/dL 5–35
Uric acid	Male 2.1–8.5 mg/dL (likely higher with age) Female 2.0–7.0 mg/dL (likely higher with age)
Vitamin A	30–65 μg/dL
White blood cell count (WBC)	4300–10,800 cells/μL/cu mm

Index

Notes: Page numbers in *italics* refer to boxes, figures and tables.

A

ABC Homeopathy, 244
abscesses, *150*
absinthe, *50, 51, 70, 122*
N-acetyl-5-
        methoxytryptamine,
        104
acetyl L-carnitine, *70, 71,
        74, 82*
acidophilus, 43–44, *70, 71,
        73, 74*
acne, 42
    herbal medicine, *73*
    homeopathic remedies,
        148, 149
aconite *see Aconitum
        napellus*
Aconitum napellus
    homeopathic symptom
        picture, *140*
    indications, *149–156*
        first aid, *157,
        158*
    safety, 136
Actaea racemosa
    homeopathic symptom
        picture, *140*
    indications, *72, 79, 150,
        152, 155*

Actea rac. *see Actaea
        racemosa*
acupressure *see
        shiatsu/acupressure*
acupuncture, 175, 178–182
    definition, 249
    indications/
        contraindications,
        3, 181
    in pregnancy, *181*
    principles, *3, 175–176,
        178–179*
        see also meridians; Qi
    web-site information,
        242
    see also shiatsu/
        acupressure
Aegle marmelos, 60
*Aesculus hippocastanum,
        71, 99*
Agathosma betulina, 72, 81
Agni, 53, 55–58, 59
Agnus castus, 72, 74
Agrimonia, 221
agrimony, *221*
AIDS, 14, *192*
Ainsworth, 134, 139, 244
alder buckthorn, *70, 92*
Alexander Technique, *3–4,*
        249
allergic reactions, *71, 81*
    to homeopathic
        medicines, 123,
        136
    rashes, *153*

Allium sativum, 36, 71, 93
Aloe barbadensis, 75
Aloe ferox, 75
aloes, *70, 73, 75*
aloe vera, *70, 72, 73, 75*
alpha-lipoic acid, *70, 73, 75*
Alternative and
        Complementary
        Medicine Directory,
        242
alternative medicine *see*
        complementary and
        alternative medicine
        (CAM)
Althaea officinalis, 71, 103
Ama, 55–58
American Academy of
        Medical Acupuncture,
        242
American Association for
        Therapeutic Humor,
        245
American Massage Therapy
        Association, 245
American Music Therapy
        Association, 246
American Society for Music
        Therapy, 246
American Society of Clinical
        Hypnosis, 245
Amla, 60
analgesia/pain management
    acupuncture, *181*
    back pain *see* back pain
    essential oils, *163*
    herbal medicine, 42
    homeopathic, *142, 145*
    hypnotherapy, 232
Ananas comosus, 72, 80
Andrographis paniculata,
        60, 70, 72
angelic acid esters, *80*
Angelica sinensis, 50, 73, 90

anise oil, *173*
anthroposophical medicine,
        33–36, 62–64
    definition, 249
    indications/
        contraindications,
        4
    mistletoe therapy, 33, 36,
        63–64
    principles, *4,* 62–63
antibacterial agents, *164*
antifungal agents, *164*
antioxidants, *73, 75, 97,*
        102
antiparasitic agents, *101*
antiseptic agents, *164*
antispasmodics, essential
        oils, *163*
anxiety, *120*
    essential oils, *164*
    homeopathic remedies,
        140, 145,
        149
    hypnotherapy, 232
Apis/Apis mel. *see Apis*
        mellifica
Apis mellifica
    homeopathic symptom
        picture, *140*
    indications, *149,*
        151–156
    first aid, *157*
appetite problems, *70,*
        149
Arctium lappa, 51
Arctostaphylos uva-ursi, 72,
        78
Argent. nit., *140, 152,*
        153
Argentum nitricum, 140,
        149, 152, 153
Aristolochia, 68, xv
arnica *see Arnica montana*

Arnica montana, 137
  homeopathic symptom
    picture, *141*
  indications, *73, 76,
    149, 150,
    152–155*
    external application,
      *72, 76, 150,
      159*
    first aid, *157, 158*
aromachology, 161
aromatherapy, 2, 160–174
  contraindications, *5*
  definition, 161, 249
  efficacy, 124–126
  indications, *5, 173–174*
  principles, *5*, 160–166
  safety, 123–124,
    161–162
  web-site information, 242
  see also essential oils
Aromatherapy Consortium,
  242
Aromatherapy Organisations
  Council (AOC), 242
aromatology, 161
Arsen. alb./Arsenicum *see*
    Arsenicum album
Arsenicum album, 149
  homeopathic symptom
    picture, *141*
  indications, *149–153,
    155, 156*
  first aid, *157, 158*
artemether, 50
Artemisia absinthium, 50,
  51, *70, 122*
Artemisia annua, 50, *51*
artemisinin, 50
arthritis, *72, 80, 85, 96,
  149*
  see also rheumatism
artichoke, 36, *70, 76*

art therapy, 2, 33, 63
  definition, 249
  indications/
    contraindications,
      5
  principles, 5
ashwagandha, 60, 61, *70,
  71, 77*
aspen, *221*
Association of Reflexologists
  (AoR), 247
Astragalus, 50, *71, 72,
  77*
Astragalus membranaceus,
  50, *71, 72, 77*
Atropa belladonna
  homeopathic symptom
    picture, *141*
  indications, *149–152,
    154–156*
  first aid, *157, 158*
  safety, 136
Autogenic Society, 242
autogenic therapy/training
  definition, 250
  indications/
    contraindications,
      6
  principles, 6
  web-site information,
    242–245
Avena sativa, *73, 105–106,
  222*
Ayurveda, 2, 52–61, 252, xii
  causes of disease in,
    58–59
  concepts/principles, 6,
    32, 52–58
    Agni, 53, 55–58,
      59
    Ama, 55–58
    Dhatus, 53, 58
    Gunas, 58

271

Ayurveda (*cont'd*)
Prakruti (human
constitution),
54, 55,
255–256
Tridosha *see* Tridosha
definition, 250
indications/
contraindications,
6
legislation, 68
treatment, 59–61, *60*,
64
Rasayana, 61

B

babies *see* children/infants
Bach, Edward, 218
see also Bach Flower
Remedies
Bach Flower Remedies, 2,
219–223, 250
administration, 222–223
emotional states,
221–222
classification, *220*
history of use, 218
indications, *7*
principles, *7*, 219–222
selection, 223
web-site information,
243
back pain
Alexander Technique,
3–4
chiropractic, *8*, 185–186,
187
osteopathy, *17*, 200, *202*
bacterial infections, *164*
bad breath, *149*
bael, 60

Balm of Gilead, *71*, 77
barberry, *70*, *72*, *78*
basil, holy, 60
basil oil, *173*
bearberry, *72*, *78*
beech, *221*
bee pollen, *70*, *78*
behavioural modification
cognitive (behavioural)
therapy, 232, 251
hypnotherapy, 230–231
bel, 60
'belief response' *see*
placebo effect/
therapy
belladonna *see Atropa
belladonna*
Bengal quince, *60*
Benveniste, Jacques, 135
benzoin oil, *162*, *173*
berberis, *70*, *72*, *78*
Berberis aquifolium, *70*, *72*,
78, *107*
bereavement, *149*
bergamot oil, *162*, *173*
beta-carotene, 44, *73*, *79*
BHMA (British Holistic
Medical Association),
241, xviii
Bhutas (Five Elements),
47–48, 53, 179
bilberry, *71*, *79*
biodynamic massage, 176
biofeedback
definition, 250
electrodermal response,
252
indications/
contraindications,
7
principles, 7
web-site information,
243

Biofeedback Foundation of Europe, 243
Biofeedback Research Bibliography, 243
bisabolol, *80*
black bryony, *159*
black cohош *see Actaea racemosa*
black haw, *72, 80*
black pepper, *60*, 61
blueberry, *71, 79*
blue green algae, *71, 117*
body humours, 40
   'Tridosha' *see* Tridosha
body odour, *150*
boils, *150*
Boiron, 244
boldo, *70, 80*
borage, *73, 118*
Borago officinalis, 73, 118
Bowen Technique, *8,* 250
breast-feeding problems, *150, 159*
British Acupuncture Council, 242
British Association of Hypnotists, 245
British Autogenic Society, 242
British College of Naturopathy and Osteopathy, 246
British College of Osteopathy, 246
British Holistic Medical Association (BHMA), 241, xviii
British Homeopathic Association, 135, *157*
British Institute of Homeopathy Ltd, 138, 244

British Medical Acupuncture Society, 242
British Naturopathic Association, 246
British School of Homeopathy, 138
British Society for Music Therapy, 246
British Society of Medical and Dental Hypnosis (BSMDH), 245
bromelain, *72, 80*
bruising
   herbal remedies, *73, 76*
   homeopathic remedies, *137, 141, 157, 159*
bryonia *see Bryonia alba*
Bryonia alba
   homeopathic symptom picture, *141*
   indications, 132, *149, 151, 153–156*
   first aid, *157*
BSMDH (British Society of Medical and Dental Hypnosis), 244
buchu, *72, 81*
burdock, *51*
burns/scalds, *97, 150, 157, 159*
butcher's broom, *71, 72, 81*
butterbur, *71, 81*

273

C

Calcarea carbonica
   indications, *141, 149, 154, 156*
Calcarea phosphorica
   homeopathic symptom picture, *142*
   indications, *154*

Calc. carb see *Calcarea carbonica*
Calc. phos see *Calcarea phosphorica*
calendula see *Calendula officinalis*
Calendula officinalis, 72, 73, 82
external application, 150, 156, 157, 158, 159
Camellia sinensis, 73, 98
camphor oil, 162, 172
cancer patients
massage and, 14, 192
mistletoe therapy, 63–64
candida infection, 74
cantharis, 142, 150, 151, 154, 156
Cantharis vesicatoria, 142, 150, 151, 154, 156
capsules, 38
caraway oil, 169, 171
Carbo veg., 142, 155
Carbo vegetabilis, 142, 155
cardamom oil, 162, 172
cardiac pacemakers, 181
cardiovascular disease, 32, 48, 71, 86, 87
L-Carnitine, 70, 71, 74, 82
carrot seed oil, 173
cascara, 70, 83
Cassia angustifolia, 70, 116
catarrh, 146, 151
cat's claw, 72, 83
centaury, 221
centella, 73, 97
Centella asiatica, 73, 97
central nervous system, 71
centring, definition, 250
Cephaelis ipecacuanha
homeopathic symptom picture, 144

indications, 150, 154, 155, 156
cerato, 221
Chamaemelum nobile, 83–84, 173
chamazulene, 80
chamomile
English or Roman see *Chamaemelum nobile*
German or Hungarian see *Matricaria recutita*
chamomilla see *Matricaria recutita*
charyita, 60
chasteberry, 72, 74
chelation therapy, 198, 251
cherry plum, 221
chestnut bud, 221
chicken pox, 147, 150
chicory, 221
chilblains, 150, 159
childbirth, 111, 154
children/infants
craniosacral therapy, 177, 202
essential oils, 171–172
homeopathic remedies, 137
chinchona bark, 81
Chinese angelica, 50, 73, 90
Chirayita, 60
chiretta, 60, 70, 72
chiropractic, 176, 185–187
definition, 251
indications/contraindications, 8, 186, 187
principles, 8, 176, 185–186, 186
regulation, 187
see also osteopathy

chitosan, 44, *70*, *84*
cholestin, *112*
chondroitin, 44, *72*, *85*
chronic fatigue syndrome, 42
  massage in, *14*, *193*
  osteopathy, 201
Chrysanthemum cinerariaefolium, *73*, *100*, *157*
Cimicifuga racemosa see Actaea racemosa
cinchona bark, *85*, 127
cinnamon bark oil, *162*, *173*
cinnamon leaf oil, 168, *173*
circle of life, 179
citronella, *173*
clary sage oil, *162*, *172*, *173*
classification (of complementary medicine), 2
claustrophobia, *150*
clematis, *221*
'clinical gaze', 23–24
cloves, *72*, *85*, *162*, *173*
coenzyme Q-10, *73*, *86*
cognitive enhancement, *71*, *74*, *94*, *164*
cognitive (behavioural) therapy
  definition, 251
  hypnotherapy and, 232
cold compresses, *199*
colds, *90*, *91*, *108*, *151*, *157*
cold sores, *146*, *151*
colic, *151*
colonic irrigation, *199*
colour therapy
  definition, 251
  indications/ contraindications, *8*
  principles, *8*

coltsfoot, *71*, *86*
complementary and alternative medicine (CAM)
  classification, 2
  definition, 251, xi–xii
  evidence base, xix–xx
  general website information, 241–242
  indications/ contraindications, *3–22*
  legal status, xvi–xvii
  media scare stories, xiv
  placebo effect and *see* placebo effect/ therapy
  qualification abbreviations, 263–269
  therapies encountered by pharmacists, 1–23, *3–22*
  website information, 241–248
  WHO guidelines, xv
  see also holistic medicine/ holism; *specific systems/therapies*
Complementary Medicine Addresses and Information, 241
Complementary Therapies in Nursing Special Interest Group (CTINSIG), xvii
concentration (lack of), *151*
cone flower, 36, *71*, *72*, *73*, *90*
consolida, *73*, *101*
constipation, *70*, *151*
consumer guidance, xv–xvi

copper ointment, *159*

coriander seed oil, *162, 172*

cough, *86, 108, 141, 143, 151*

counselling, *9*, 251, 256

crab apple, *221*

cramp, *142, 151, 157, 159*

cramp bark, *72, 86*

cranberry, *72, 87*

craniosacral therapy, 177, 202

Crataegus oxyacanthoides, 36, 71, 98

creatine, *70, 87*

crystal therapy, 2
   definition, 251
   indications/
       contraindications, 9
   principles, 9

CTINSIG (Complementary Therapies in Nursing Special Interest Group), xvii

Cucurbita pepo, 73, 109

Cuprum met., *142, 151*

Cuprum metallicum, 142, 151

Curcuma longa, 36, 70, 71, 72, 73, 119

cuts/grazes, *158, 159*

Cynara scolymus, 36, 70, 76

cystitis, 42, *81, 87, 142, 151*

decongestants, essential oils, *164*

deep brain stimulation, placebo effect, 29

dehydroepiandrosterone (DHEA), *72, 73, 89*

Delphinium consolida, 73, 101

Delphinium staphisagria, 147, 149, 151, 155

dementia, *94*
   music therapy, 236, *237*

Demystifying Homeopathy, 244

dental treatment, *152*

Department of Complementary Therapies, 139

depression, *4*, 42
   herbal remedies, *71, 114*
   homeopathic remedies, *140, 147, 152*

detoxification, 60, 197, 198

devil's claw, *72, 88*

DHA (docosahexaenoic acid), *71, 72, 89*

Dhatus, 53, 58

DHEA (dehydroepiandro-sterone), *72, 73, 89*

diabetes, *51, 75, 110*

diarrhoea, *74, 97, 152*

digestive problems *see* gastrointestinal/digestive problems

dill oil, 169, *173*

Dioscorea villosa, 72, 73, 121

docosahexaenoic acid (DHA), *72, 89, 711*

Dong Quai, 50, *73, 90*

Doshas, 53, 252
   see also Kapha; Pitta; Vata

D

dandelion, *71, 88*

dandruff, *143, 151, 159*

Dang Gui, 50, *73, 90*

Dan Shen, 50, *71, 87*

decoctions, *37*

Drosera, *143, 154*
Drosera rotundifolia, 143, 154
drug addiction, hypnotherapy, 217
drug interactions, 1
    essential oils, 123, 174
    herbal supplements, 33–34, *70–118*
    homeopathic remedies, 123, 136
dysmenorrhoea, *80, 86, 90, 141, 145, 165*
dyspepsia, *70*

E

earache, *152*
ear infections, *146*
Echinacea, 36, 71, 72, 73, 90
eczema, 42
    herbal remedies, *73, 91*
    homeopathic remedies, *143, 152, 159*
EDR (electrodermal response), 252
EDTA (ethylene diamine tetraacetic acid), 198
efficacy, xix–xx
effleurage, *191*
eicosapentaenoic acid (EPA), 89
elderberry, 36, 71, 72, 91
elderflower, 36, 71, 72, 91
electrodermal response (EDR), 252
Eleutherococcus senticocus, 71, 95
elm, *221*
emotional/psychological therapies, 217–239

see also specific therapies
empathy, 23
endocrine problems *see hormonal problems*
enemas, *199*
EPA (eicosapentaenoic acid), 89
Ephedra sinica, 71, 103
epilepsy, essential oils and, 172
essential oils, 2
    administration routes, 169–170
    allergic reaction, 123
    children, 171–172
    chirality, 167
    definition, 252
    drug interactions, 123, 174
    formulation, 170–171
    gender differences, 168–169
    indications, 165, 166, 171–172, *173–174*
    pharmacological activities, *163–166*
    pregnancy, *162, 172*
    quality, 167–168
    safety, 123–124, *161–162*, 167–168
    synergy and quenching, 168
    see also aromatherapy
ether, 53
ethical considerations, placebos, 26–27
ethylene diamine tetraacetic acid (EDTA), 198
eucalyptus oil, 171, *173*

Eugenia caryophyllata, 72, 85, 162, 173
Euphrasia, 143, 151, 152
Euphrasia officinalis, 143, 151, 152
eurythmy, 33, 63
evening primrose, 73, 91, 159
examination nerves, 152
exhaustion, 152
expectorants, essential oils, 164
eyebright, 143, 151, 152
eye inflammation/infection, 143, 152

F

Faculty of Homeopathy Academic Department, Glasgow Homeopathic Hospital, 244
Faculty of Homeopathy London, 244
fasting, 198
fatigue, 51, 113
fear, 152
fennel oil, 169, 173
Ferr phos., 143, 153
Ferrum phosphoricum, 143, 153
fever, 49–50, 51, 131–132, 141
feverfew, 72, 91
Filipendula ulmaria, 72, 103
first aid, homeopathic, 137, 157–158
fish oils, 71, 72, 89
Fitzgerald, William, 205

Five Elements (Bhutas), 47–48, 53, 179
flavonoids, 80
flaxseed, 71, 73, 92
flu, 151
Food Act (1990), 68
food poisoning, 141, 152, 156
foods, functional *see* nutraceuticals
fractures, 147, 149, 158
frangula, 70, 92
frankincense oil, 173
functional foods *see* nutraceuticals
fungal infections, 164

G

Ganoderma lucidum, 50
garlic, 36, 71, 93
gastrointestinal/digestive problems
    constipation, 146
    diarrhoea, 147, 152
    essential oils, 163–164, 169
    food poisoning, 141, 152, 156
    herbal remedies, 41, 64, 70, 82, 108
    homeopathic remedies, 142, 144, 158
    irritable bowel syndrome, 41
    nausea/vomiting *see* nausea/vomiting
Gattefosse, Rene-Maurice, 161
Gelsemium *see Gelsemium sempervirens*

Gelsemium sempervirens
    indications, *143, 149,
        152-154*
    first aid, *157, 158*
gender differences, essential
        oils, 168-169
General Council and
        Register of
        Naturopaths, 246
General Osteopathic
        Council, 201, 246
gentian, *70, 93,* 221
*Gentiana lutea, 70, 93,
        221*
geopathic stress, 2
    definition, 252
    principles, *11*
geranium oil, *162,* 172
giddiness, *153*
ginger, 36, *51,* 64-65, *70,
        94*
ginger oil, *162,* 172
ginkgo, 36, 39, *71,* 94
*Ginkgo biloba, 36, 39, 71,
        94*
ginseng
    American, *95*
    Korean, 50, *51, 70, 71,
        95*
    Siberian, *71, 95*
glucosamine, *72, 96*
Glycine max, 73, 117
Glycyrrhiza glabra, 70, 101
Glycyrrhiza uralensis, 101
golden rod, *72, 96*
goldenseal, *70, 72, 97*
gorse, *221*
gotu kola, *73, 97*
gout, *153*
grapeseed, *73, 97*
Graphites, *143, 152, 155,
        159*
grazes/cuts, *156*

green chiretta, *60, 70, 72*
green tea, *73, 98*
grief, *146, 149*
guarana, *70, 71, 98*
Guided imagery, 247
Gunas, 58

H

haemorrhoids (piles), *71, 79,
        81, 148, 153, 159*
Hahnemann Academy of
        Homeopathy, 139
Hahnemann, Samuel,
        127-128
Hahnemann's principles,
        133
halitosis, *149*
Hamamelis, *153, 159*
Hara diagnosis, 213
    definition, 252
    indications/
        contraindications,
        11
    principles, *11*
*Harpagophytum
        procumbens, 72, 88*
hawthorn, 36, *71, 98*
hayfever, *71, 81, 97, 143,
        146*
headaches
    chiropractic, 186
    herbal remedies, *72,
        91*
    homeopathic remedies,
        142, 153
    placebo therapy, 27
    reflexology, 206-207
head lice, *73, 100*
healing, 224-226
    approaches, *226*
        stages, *227*

healing (*cont'd*)
  *see also specific
      approaches*
  definition, 218, 252
  indications, *227*
  principles, *10,* 224–226
'healing crisis,' 208
heart disease, 32, *48, 71*
heart pacemakers, *181*
heather, *221*
heatstroke, *156, 158*
Helios, 138, 139, 244
Helsinki Declaration, 27
Hepar sulph., *144, 149,
      150, 152, 155*
*Hepar sulphuris, 144, 149,
      150, 152, 155*
herbal medicine, 31–122
  anthrosophical medicine
        see
        anthroposophical
        medicine
  Ayurveda *see* Ayurveda
  contraindications,
        74–122
  definition, 252
  doses, *74–122*
  drug interactions, 33–34,
        74–122
  evidence-based (rational
        phytotherapy),
        31–32, 36, 40–42,
        64
  food-based
        (nutraceuticals) *see*
        nutraceuticals
  indications, *10,* 41–42,
        70–122
  licensing issues, 66–68
  preparation forms,
        37–38
  prescriptions, 42
  principles, *10*

  quality, 38–39
  regulation, 66–68,
        66–72
  self-medication, 42
  Traditional Chinese *see*
        Traditional
        Chinese Medicine
        (TCM)
  Traditional Western, 31,
        40–42
  treatment choice, 65
  web-site information,
        243
  *see also specific
        supplements/
        medicines*
hives, *153*
holistic medicine/holism,
      23–25
  'clinical gaze' and, 23–24
  definition, 23, 252–253
  'pharmaceutical gaze,'
        24–25
  website information, 248
holly, *221*
holy basil, 60
Homeopathic Medical
      Association, 244
homeopathy, 2, 123–159
  allergic reactions to, 123,
        136
  children, 137
  concepts/principles, *11,*
        127–130
    like cures like,
          128–129, 253
    potentization
          concept,
          129–130
    single *vs.* multiple
          remedies, 130
  contraindications, *11*
  definition, 253

dose and preparation,
129–130, 132, 134
drug interactions, 123,
136
fficacy, 124, 135
external application,
137, *159*
first aid, 137, *157–158*
indications, *11*,
144–151,
148–148
institutions/professional
bodies, 138
manufacturers/suppliers,
139
'mother tinctures,' 141
patterns of use, *125*
pharmacists' role, 133
dispensing, 134
placebo effect, 124
safety, 136
'symptom pictures,' 128,
130–131
remedy matching,
131, 148–148
training courses, 139
web-site information,
243–244
see also Bach Flower
Remedies; *specific
remedies*
honeysuckle, *221*
hops, *71, 99*
hormonal problems
essential oils, *165,
174*
herbal remedies, 42,
72–73
homeopathic remedies,
147
hornbeam, *221*
horse-chestnut, *71, 99*
hot compresses, *199*

human constitution,
Ayurvedic medicine
see Prakruti (human
constitution)
humour and laughter
therapy, 2
definition, 253
indications/
contraindications,
12
principles, *12*
web-site information,
245
Humulus lupulus, 71, 99
*Hydrastis canadensis, 70,
72, 97*
hydrocotyle, *73, 97*
hydrotherapy, *199*
3 hydroxy 4 *N*
trimethylaminobutyric
acid, *70, 71, 82*
hypercholesterolaemia, *71,
93*
Hypericum *see Hypericum
perforatum*
Hypericum perforatum, 149,
xix–xx
dosage, *110*
drug interactions, *110*
homeopathic symptom
picture, *144*
indications, *72, 114,
149, 152–153,
155*
external application,
*73, 157, 158,
159*
licensing issues, 36
hypertension, *4, 48, 71, 87,*
232
hypnotherapy, 217, 230–233
contraindications, *12,
233*

hypotherapy (cont'd)
definition, 218, 253
indications, *12, 217, 232, 233*
principles, *12,* 230–231
stages, *232*
web-site information, 245
hyssop oil, *162,* 172, *173*

I

Ignatia, *144, 149, 152, 153*
Ignatia amara, 144, 149, 152, 153
impatiens, *221*
Indian gooseberry, *60,* 61
Indian pennywort, *73, 97*
infants *see* children/infants
infection/infectious diseases, *72*
essential oils, *164*
see also specific conditions
influenza, *90, 91, 143, 151, 155*
injuries, 137, *149*
Innerself, 247
insect bites/stings
essential oils, *165*
homeopathic remedies, *149, 157, 159*
insect flowers, *73, 100, 157*
insomnia, *120,* 177
acupuncture, *181*
essential oils, *165–166*
homeopathic remedies, *140, 141*
hypnotherapy, 232
Institute of Complementary Medicine, 241
integrated medicine, 251

see also complementary and alternative medicine (CAM)
International Council of Reflexologists, 247
International Federation of Aromatherapists, 242
International Veterinary Acupuncture Association, 242
Ipecac *see Cephaelis ipecacuanha*
iridology
definition, 253
indications/contraindications, *13*
principles, *13*
irritable bowel syndrome, 41, *70*
Iscador M, 64
Iscador P, 64
Iscador Qu, 64

J

jasmine oil, *162,* 172
Jesuit's bark, *85,* 127
jet-lag, *154*
jiu (moxibustion), 177, 254

K

Kali. bich., *145, 150, 151, 153, 156*
Kalium bichromicum, 145, 150, 151, 153, 156
Kalmegh, 60
Kalmirch, 60
Kapha, 32, 53–55, 59
constitution, *54*

food effects, *56–57*
herb effects, *60*
Kaposi's sarcoma, *14*, *192*
karma, *59*
kava-kava, *100*
Ki *see* Qi
kinesiology, *13*, *253–254*

L

labour pains, *154*
Lachesis *see Lachesis muta muta*
Lachesis muta muta
    homeopathic symptom picture, *145*
    indications, *132*, *149*, *151*, *154*
lactation problems, *150*, *157*
Lactobacillus acidophilus, *43–44*, *70*, *71*, *73*, *74*
Lactuca virosa, *71*, *101*
lapacho, *100*
larch, *221*
larkspur, *73*, *101*
laryngitis, *86*, *154*
laughter therapy *see* humour and laughter therapy
laurel oil, *162*
lavender oil, *162*, *172*, *173*
Law of Similars (like cures like), *128–129*, *253*
legal status (of complementary medicine), *xiv–xv*
lemon balm, *71*, *72*, *101*, *173*
lemon oil, *173*
Le Shan, *226*
lettuce, *71*, *101*
lettuce opium, *71*, *101*

licorice, *70*, *101*
D-limonene, *167*
linseed, *71*, *73*, *92*
Linum usitatissimum, *71*, *73*, *88*
liquid extracts, *37*
liquorice, *70*, *101*
lycopene, *44*, *73*, *102*
Lycopodium, *145*, *149*, *151–154*, *156*
Lycopodium clavatum, *145*, *149*, *151–154*, *156*

M

Mahonia aquifolium, *70*, *72*, *107*
Ma Huang, *71*, *103*
malaria, *51*, *127*
marigold *see Calendula officinalis*
marjoram oil, *173*
Marrubium vulgare, *71*, *121*
marshmallow, *71*, *103*
massage, *175*, *189–191*
    chronic fatigue syndrome, *14*, *193*
    definition, *254*
    indications/contraindications, *14*
    movements, *191*
    principles, *14*, *176*, *189–190*
    Swedish, *14*, *176*, *189–190*, *257*
    web-site information, *245*
    see also specific types/ approaches
Mathie, Robert, *135*

Matricaria recutita
external use, *79–80,*
159, 173
homeopathic symptom
picture, *142*
indications, *83, 151,*
152, 154–156
Maury, Marguerite, 161
meadowsweet, *72, 103*
measles, *154*
media scare stories, xiv
Medline, 248
Medline plus, 243
Melaleuca alternifolia
indications, *72, 73, 118,*
159, 170, *174*
safety, *161,* 167–168
melatonin, *104*
Melissa officinalis, 71, 72,
101, 173
memory enhancement, *94,*
113, 115, 164
menopause, 42, 74, 79, 90,
92
essential oils, *165*
homeopathic remedies,
146, 147, 154
menstrual problems, 74,
80
dysmenorrhoea, *80, 86,*
90, 141, 145,
165
homeopathic remedies,
154
see also premenstrual
syndrome
Mentha piperita, 70, 109,
169, 171, *174*
menthol, *71*
Merc. sol, *145, 149, 150,*
152–156
Mercury, *145, 149, 150,*
152–156

meridians, 180
definition, 179, 254
in shiatsu, *212, 213*
migraine *see* headaches
milk thistle, *70, 104*
mimulus, *221*
mistletoe therapy, 33, 36,
63–64
Monascus purpureus, 112
monkshood *see Aconitum*
napellus
morning sickness, 180, 213
'mother tinctures,' 132
mountain grape, *70, 72, 107*
mountain tobacco *see*
Arnica montana
mouth ulcers, *85, 145,*
154
moxibustion (jiu), 177, 254
mugwort, 180
multiple sclerosis, *75*
Multiple Sclerosis Society,
247
mumps, *155*
musculoskeletal problems
chiropractic *see*
chiropractic
osteopathy *see*
osteopathy
physical therapy, 175
music therapy, 218,
236–238
contraindications, *15*
definition, 218, 254
indications, *15, 238*
precautions, *238*
principles, *15*
web-site information,
246
mustard, *221*
Myroxylon balsamum, 71,
72, 119
myrrh oil, *173*

N

nappy rash, *159*
National Center for
        Complementary and
        Alternative Medicine,
        224–225
National Center for
        Complementary and
        Alternative Medicine:
        Complementary and
        Alternative Medicine
        in the US, 241
National Federation of
        Spiritual Healers
        (NFSH), 248
National Institute of Medical
        Herbalists, 243
National Register of
        Hypnotherapists and
        Psychotherapists, 245
Nat. mur., *146, 151, 153,
        154, 156*
*Natrum muriacatum, 146,
        151, 153, 154, 156*
naturopathy, 196–199
        definition, 254
        indications/
                contraindications,
                15
        pregnancy, 196, *198*
        principles, *15*, 176,
                196–197
        safety, 198–199
        web-site information,
                246
nausea/vomiting
        acupressure bands, 177,
                179–180, 211,
                213
        herbal remedies, *70, 94*
        homeopathic remedies,
                142, 144, 156

morning sickness, 180,
        213
travel sickness *see* travel
        sickness
Nelsons Homeopathy and
        Bach Flower
        Remedies, 139
        web-site information,
                134, 138, 244
neroli oil, *162, 172, 173*
nettle, *73, 105*
neurolinguistic
        programming, *16,*
        254–255
nicotine replacement
        therapy, placebo
        effect, 29
nocebo effect, 25–26, 27–29
        see also placebo effect/
                therapy
nosebleeds, *155*
nutraceuticals, 32, 43–44
        definition, 43, 252, 255
        indications/
                contraindications,
                16
        principles, *16*
        product quality, 38–39
        treatment choice, 65
        *see also specific
                supplements*
Nux vom.
        homeopathic symptom
                picture, *146*
        indications, 136, *151,
                153, 154, 156*
        first aid, *157, 158*

O

oak, *221*
oats, *73, 105–106, 222*

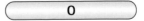

Ocimum sanctum, 60
octosanol, 44, *70, 71, 106*
Oenothera biennis, 73, 91,
          159
olive, *221*
Omega-3-fatty acids, *89*
oragano oil, *173*
orange oil, *174*
Oregon grape, *70, 72, 107*
ornithine alpha
          ketoglutarate, *70, 73,*
          107
osteopathy, 175, 200–203
    contraindications, *17*
    definition, *255*
    indications, *17*, 201, *202*
    passive palpatory
          examination,
          201–202
    precautions, *203*
    principles, *17*, 177,
          200–201
    regulation, *187*
    web-site information,
          246
    see also chiropractic
osteoporosis, *22, 203, 211*

pacemakers, *181*
pain management *see*
          analgesia/pain
          management
palpation, 201–202
panaceas, *61*
Panax ginseng, 50, 51, *70,*
          71, 95
Panax notoginseng, 95
Panax pseudoginseng, 95
Panax quinquefolius, 95
Panchakarma, 60

Parkinson's disease, placebo
          response, 27–28
parsley oil, *162, 172*
passiflora, 36, *108*
Passiflora incarnate, 36,
          108
passionflower, 36, 108
patchouli oil, *162, 172, 174*
pau d'arco, *100*
Paullinia cupana, *70, 71, 98*
pelargonium, *72, 108*
Pelargonium sidioides, *72,*
          108
peppermint, *70*, 109, 169,
          171, *174*
peppermint oil, *71, 105*
percussion, *191*
Petasites vulgaris, *71, 81*
petitgrain oil, *162, 174*
petrissage, *191*
Peumus boldo, *70, 80*
'pharmaceutical gaze,' 24–25
pharmacists
    'pharmaceutical gaze,'
          24–25
    role in homeopathy, 133
    therapies encountered
          by, *1–23, 3–22*
    see also specific
          therapies
Phosphorus, *146, 150, 153,*
          154, 155
Phyllanthus emblica, *60*, 61
physical therapies, 175–215
    see also specific
          therapies
phytochemicals, 43–44
    see also herbal medicine;
          nutraceuticals
phytotherapy *see* herbal
          medicine
piles (haemorrhoids), *71, 79,*
          148, 153, 157

pine, *110, 162, 174, 221*
pineapple enzymes, *72, 80*
pine bark extract, *71, 73, 110*
Pinus maritima, 71, 73, 110
Piper longum, 60, 61
Piper methysticum, 100
Pitta, 32, 53–55, 59, 252, 258
    constitution, *54*
    food effects, *56–57*
    herb effects, *60*
placebo effect/therapy, 25–29
    contraindications, *17*
    definition, 25–26, *255*
    efficacy, 27
    ethical considerations, 26–27
    herbal medicine, 36
    homeopathy and, 124
    negative (nocebo) effect, 25–26, 27–29
    principles, *17*
polarity therapy, *255*
policosanol, 44, *70, 71, 106*
poplar buds, *71, 77*
Populus, 71, 77
postnatal care, *155*
Potter's Herbal Medicines, 243
Prakruti (human constitution), *54, 55, 255–256*
Prana, 53, *256*
pregnancy
    acupuncture in, *181*
    essential oils, *162, 172*
    massage in, *14, 193*
    morning sickness, 180, 213
    naturopathy and, 196, *198*
    reflexology, *18, 205*

premenstrual syndrome (PMS), 42, *91,* 206
    essential oils, *165*
    homeopathic remedies, *141, 154*
prescriptions/prescribing
    CAM interactions with prescribed drugs
        see drug interactions
    herbal medicines, 42
    homeopathic remedies, 134
Prince of Wales's Foundation for Integrated Health, 241, xviii
probiotics, 43–44, *70*
professional registering bodies, xviii–xix
        see also specific organisations
Prunus africana, 73, 110
psoriasis, *51, 107, 155, 159*
psychological/emotional therapies *see specific therapies*
Pulsatilla, *146, 149–156*
Pulsatilla nigricans, 146, 149–156
pulse diagnosis, 49
pumpkin seed, *73, 109*
pycnogenol, *71, 73, 97, 110*
Pygeum africanum, 73, 110
pygeum bark, *73, 110*
pyrethrum, *73, 100, 159*

Q

Qi, 32, 46–50, 53, 180
    acupuncture and, 176
    definition, *256*

Qi (*cont'd*)
    reflexology and, 207
    shiatsu and, 211
Qi-Gong
    definition, 256
    principles, *17*
queen of the meadow, 72,
    103
quenching, essential oils,
    168

R

randomised clinical trials
    (RCTs)
    homeopathy, 135–136
    reflexology, 206
Rasayana, 61
raspberry leaf, *73, 111*
rational phytotherapy,
    31–32, 36, 40–42, 64
    see also herbal medicine
red chestnut, *221*
red clover, *73, 111*
red vine leaf, *73, 93, 112*
red yeast rice, *112*
reflexology, 175, 205–209
    benefits, *208*
    contraindications, *18,*
        209
    definition, 256
    'healing crisis,' 208
    indications, *18,* 206–207
    pregnancy, *18,* 205
    principles, *18,* 177,
        205–207
    see also Qi
    web-site information,
        247
reiki, 2, 224, *226*
    definition, 256
    indications/

contraindications,
    18
    principles, *18*
Reishi mushroom, 50
relaxation, *19,* 247,
    256–257
remedies (homeopathic) *see*
    homeopathy
'reproductive-metabolic'
    system, 62–63
'Rescue Remedy,' 218,
    219–222, *220,* 223
research, 1, xix–xx
    see also randomised
        clinical trials
        (RCTs); *specific*
        therapies
Research Council for
    Complementary
    Medicine, 241
respiratory conditions
    cough, *86, 108, 141,*
        151
    essential oils, *164–165,*
        169, 171
    herbal remedies, 42, *71,*
        119
    influenza, *90, 91, 143,*
        151, 155
    see also specific
        conditions
Rhamnus frangula, 70, 92
Rhamnus purshianus, 70,
    83
Rheum, 70, 113
rheumatism
    herbal remedies, *72, 88,*
        119
    homeopathic remedies,
        147, 155, 159
    see also arthritis
rhodiola, *70, 71, 113*
Rhodiola rosea, 70, 71, 113

rhubarb, *70, 113*
Rhus tox.
    homeopathic symptom
        picture, *147*
    indications, *150, 152,
        153, 155, 156*
        external application,
            159
        first aid, *157, 158*
Rhus toxicodendron see
    Rhus tox.
'rhythmic' system, 63
rock rose, *221*
rock water, *221*
rosemary, *71, 113, 162,
    174*
rose oil, *162, 172, 174*
*Rosmarinus officinalis, 71,
    113, 162, 174*
Royal Pharmaceutical
    Society of Great
    Britain (RPSGB),
    xvi–xvii
Rubus ideaeus, 73, 111
rue oil, *162*
Ruscus aculeatus, 71, 72, 81
Ruta grav., *147, 152, 155,
    159*
*Ruta graveolens, 147, 150,
    152, 157*

S

sabal, *73, 115*
Sabal serrulata, 73, 115
Sacred Space Foundation,
    248
safety issues
    essential oils, 123–124,
        161–162,
        167–168
    homeopathy, 136

naturopathy, *198–199*
    see also drug interactions
sage, *71, 72, 115, 162, 172,
    174*
Salix alba, 72, 122, 222
*Salvia lavandulifolia, 71,
    115, 162, 172, 174*
*Salvia miltiorrhiza, 50, 71,
    87*
*Salvia officinalis, 71, 72,
    115, 162, 172, 174*
*Sambucus nigra, 36, 71, 72,
    91*
sandalwood oil, *162, 172,
    174*
savory oil, *162*
saw palmetto, *73, 115*
scabies, *100*
scalds see burns/scalds
scars/scarring, essential oils,
    166
schisandra, *70, 116*
*Schisandra chinensis, 70,
    116*
sciatica, *155*
scleranthus, *221*
sedatives, essential oils, *165*
self-medication, herbal
    medicine, 42
senna, *70, 116*
'sense-nervous' system, 62
Sepia, *147, 150, 152, 154*
Serenoa repens, 73, 115
Seven Emotions, 49
shamanism, 224, 225–226,
    226
    see also healing
shiatsu/acupressure, 175,
    211–213
    contraindications, *20,
        213*
    definition, 257
    diagnosis, 213, *214*

shiatsu/acupressure (*cont'd*)
 indications, *20, 212*
  travel sickness, 177,
   179–180, 211,
   213
 meridians, 212, 213
 principles, *20*, 177,
  179–180, 211–212
 web-site information,
  247
 see also acupuncture
Shiatsu Society, 247
shingles, *155*
Silica, *147, 149–150,
  155–156*
Silybum marianum, 70, 104
sinusitis, *71, 145, 156*
Six Excesses, 49
skin conditions, *73, 107,
  159, 174*
 *see also specific
  conditions*
slimming aids, *80, 84, 103*
smoking cessation
 hypnotherapy, 217, 231,
  232
 nicotine replacement
  therapy, 29
Society of Homeopaths,
  138–139, 244
Solidago virgaurea, 72, 96
solid extracts, *37*
sore throat, *145, 156*
soya, *73, 117*
soya isoflavones, 44
'Spanish fly,' *142, 150, 151,
  154, 156*
spinal manipulation therapy
  (SMT), 186
 see also chiropractic
Spiraea filipendula, 72, 103
spiritual healing, 224, 225,
  226, 248

spirulina, *71, 117*
*Spirulina platensis, 71,
  117*
splinters, *156*
sprains/strains, *147, 158,
  159*
Staphisagria, *147, 149,
  151, 155*
star anise oil, *173*
starflower, *73, 118*
Star of Bethlehem, *221*
stavesacre, *147, 149, 151,
  155*
Steiner, Rudolf, 62
stimulants, *71, 166*
St John's wort *see
  Hypericum
  perforatum*
St Mary's thistle, *70, 104*
stone therapy, *9*
 see also crystal therapy
Strychnos nux vomica see
  Nux. vom
succussion, 257
Sulphur, *148, 150, 152,
  155*
sunburn, *142, 156, 157*
Swedish massage, *14*, 176,
  189–190, 257
sweet chestnut, *222*
sweet wormwood, 50, *51*
Swertia chirata, 60
synergy, essential oils,
  168
*Syzygium aromaticum, 72,
  85, 162, 173*

T

Tabebuia avellanedae, 100
tablets, *38*
taget oil, *162*

taheebo, *100*

Tai Chi, *20, 22*, 257

Tamus, *159*

Tanacetum parthenium, *72, 91*

tapotement, *191*

Taraxacum officinale, *71, 88*

teas/infusions, *37*
  Camellia sinensis (green tea), *94*

tea tree oil *see Melaleuca alternifolia*

teething problems, *141, 142, 156*

therapeutic touch (TT), *21, 248*, 257

thioctic acid, *70, 73, 75*

thirst, *156*

TIIMPD (Traditional Herbal Medicinal Product Directive), 67

Thuja, *148, 150, 156*

Thuja occidentalis, *148, 150, 156*

thyme, *71, 72, 118*, 162, 171, *174*

Thymus vulgaris, *71, 72, 118*, 162, 171, *174*

tiger bones, 45

tiglic acid esters, *80*

tinctures, *38*

Tisserand, Robert, 161

tolu balsam, *71, 72, 119*

toothache, *85, 141, 156, 157, 159*

Traditional Chinese Medicine (TCM), 2, 45–50, xii
  causes of disease in, 49
  concepts/development, 32, 45–49, *47, 48*

Five Elements (Bhutas), 47–48, 53, 179
  Qi *see* Qi
  yin and yang *see* yin/yang
  definition, 257
  legislation, 68
  principles, *21*
  treatment in, 47–50, *51*, 64

Traditional Herbal Medicinal Product Directive (THMPD), 67

Traditional (Western) medical herbalism, 31, 40–42

trance, 257
  see also hypnotherapy

travel sickness
  homeopathic remedies, *144, 146, 156*
  shiatsu, 177, 179–180, 211, 213

Tridosha, 32, 52, 53–59
  definition, 258
  food effects, 56–57
  herb effects, 60
  human constitution determination, 54
  humours, 52, 53–55
    Kapha *see* Kapha
    Pitta *see* Pitta
    Vata *see* Vata

Trifolium pratense, *73, 111*

triterpenes, *102*

tsubos, 180, 212, 213, 254

tui na, 212

tulsi, *60*

turmeric, 36, *70, 71, 72, 73, 119*

Tussilago farfara, *71, 86*

U

Umckaloabo, *72, 108*
Una de gato, *72, 83*
unani-tibb *see* Ayurveda
Uncaria species, 72, 83
Urtica dioica, 73, 105
Urtica ointment, *157, 159*
urticaria, *153*
uva-ursi, *72, 78*

V

Vaccinium macrocarpon, 72, 87
Vaccinium myrtillus, 71, 79
Vaccinium oxycoccus, 72, 87
vaginal infections, *170*
valerian, *34, 71, 120*
Valeriana officinalis, 34, 71, 120
Valnet, Jean, *161*
Vata, *32, 53–55, 58–59, 252, 258*
    constitution, *54*
    food effects, *56–57*
    herb effects, *60*
verbena, *71, 120, 162, 222*
Verbena officinalis, 71, 116, 162, 222
vertigo, *140, 153*
vervain, *71, 120, 162, 222*
Viburnum opulus, 72, 86
Viburnum prunifolium, 72, 80
vine, *222*
visualization, *21, 247, 258*
Vital Organs, *47–48, 48*
Vitex agnus castus, 72, 74
Vitis vinifera, 73, 97, 112

vomiting *see* nausea/vomiting

W

walnut, *222*
warts, *148, 156*
water violet, *222*
website information, *241–247*
Weleda Ltd, *139, 243*
white chestnut, *222*
white horehound, *71, 121*
WHO guidelines, *xv*
wild oat, *73, 101–102, 222*
wild rose, *222*
wild yam, *72, 73, 121*
willow, *72, 122, 222*
willow bark, *72, 117, 222*
winter cherry, *60, 61, 70, 71, 77*
Withania somnifera, 60, 61, 70, 71, 77
wormwood, *50, 51, 70, 122*
wounds, *144, 149, 156, 159, 166*
wristbands, nausea treatment, *177, 179–180, 211, 213*

Y

yin/yang, *32, 45–50, 47, 180*
    definition, *258*
yoga, *22, 258*

Z

Zingiber officinalis, 36, 51, 64–65, 70, 94